1999
MUTUAL FUNDS AND RRSPs ONLINE

Jim Carroll
Rick Broadhead

**Prentice Hall Canada Inc.
Scarborough, Ontario**

Canadian Cataloguing in Publication Data

Carroll, Jim, 1959–
1999 Mutual funds and RRSPs online

2nd ed.
Previous edition published under title: Mutual funds and RRSPs online.
ISBN 0-13-974999-3

1. Finance, Personal—Canada—Computer network resources. 2. Internet (Computer network). 3. World Wide Web (Information retrieval system).
I. Broadhead, Rick.   II. Title.   III. Title: Mutual funds and RRSPs online.

HF179.C297 1999   332.024'00285'467   C99-932065-0

  © 1999 J.A. Carroll and Rick Broadhead

ALL RIGHTS RESERVED

No part of this book may be reproduced in any form without permission in writing from the publisher.

Prentice-Hall, Inc., Upper Saddle River, New Jersey
Prentice-Hall International (UK) Limited, London
Prentice-Hall of Australia, Pty. Limited, Sydney
Prentice-Hall Hispanoamericana, S.A., Mexico City
Prentice-Hall of India Private Limited, New Delhi
Prentice-Hall of Japan, Inc., Tokyo
Simon & Schuster Southeast Asia Private Limited, Singapore
Editora Prentice-Hall do Brasil, Ltda., Rio de Janeiro

ISBN 0-13-974999-3

Director, Trade and Marketing: Robert Harris
Copy Editor: Betty R. Robinson
Production Editor: Avivah Wargon
Editorial Assistant: Joan Whitman
Production Coordinator: Shannon Potts
Art Director: Mary Opper
Cover Design: Sputnik
Cover Image: Andre Baranowski/Graphistock
Page Layout: Jack Steiner

1 2 3 4 5 W 03 02 01 00 99

Printed and bound in Canada.

Neither the publisher nor author is rendering professional or legal advice in this book. If such assistance is required, the services of a qualified professional should be sought. Every effort has been made to ensure that the resources listed in this book were correct at the time of printing. Neither the author nor the publisher shall be liable for any errors or omissions in data, nor for any damages that may occur from the use of any resource contained in this book.

Visit the Prentice Hall Canada Web site! Send us your comments, browse our catalogues, and more: **www.phcanada.com**

CONTENTS

Conventions Used in This Book *vi*
Acknowledgments *vii*
About the Authors *viii*
Your Experiences with Online Finance *x*

Chapter 1—Investing on the Internet *1*
Survey After Survey... *3*
You Do Not Have to Be a Brilliant Computer Geek to Read This Book *6*

Chapter 2—The Benefits and Risks of Using the Internet for Online Investing *7*
The Benefits of Using the Internet for Your Retirement and Investment Decisions *9*
The Risks of Using the Internet as an Investment Tool *12*
Evaluating the Credibility and Validity of Online Information *33*
Where to Get Help *38*

Chapter 3—Determining What to Invest In *41*
Everyone Has a Theory *42*
The Need for Diversification! *44*
Educate Yourself *45*
Asset Mix *48*
Your Investment Objectives *55*
Figuring Our Your Asset Mix *56*
The Role of the Internet with Your Investments *57*

Chapter 4—Using Financial Calculators *59*
Five Important Financial Questions *60*
The Emergence of Sophisticated Planning Tools *67*
Two Final Hints *69*

CONTENTS

Chapter 5—Cash and Cash-Equivalent Investments on the Internet 71
Using the Internet to Compare Savings Rates 72
Understanding Innovative Product Offerings 73
Learning About the Security of Your Investment 76
Conclusion 80

Chapter 6—Mutual Funds on the Internet 81
Researching Specific Mutual Funds on the Internet 82
Online Discussion Forums 91
Making a Decision 93

Chapter 7—Researching Stocks and Bonds on the Internet 95
Using the Internet for Company Research 96
Conclusion 107

Chapter 8—Online Investing 109
Discount Brokers on the Internet 110
Researching Internet-Based Online Trading Services 111
Commissions and Fees 116
An Example of Online Trading 122
Continuing to Learn About Online Trading 125
The Future? 129

Chapter 9—Monitoring Your Performance 133
Cash-Based Investments 134
Mutual Funds 138
Stocks 153
The Future of Investment Tracking Online 162
The Bottom Line 168

Chapter 10—Don't Become Overconfident 171
The Reality? 172

Appendix A—Learning About the Basics of Retirement Planning and RRSPs on the Internet 175
Retirement Planning 176
Summary 193

Appendix B—Basic Investment Concepts 197
Do You Know What Type of Investor You Are? 198
Types of Financial Investments 202
The Role of the Internet in Investing 209

Appendix C—Mutual Fund Concepts *211*
Mutual Fund Basics *212*
What Mutual Funds Invest In *216*
The Pros and Cons of Mutual Funds *223*
What It Comes Down To *226*

Appendix D—Learning About Investments on the Internet *229*
Learning About Cash-Based Investments Online *229*
Learning About Mutual Funds Online *233*
Learning More About the Stock Market and Other Investments Online *238*
Conclusion *243*

Index *245*

CONVENTIONS USED IN THIS BOOK

To access the resources listed in this book, you will need to have access to the Internet and know how to use basic Internet tools such as the World Wide Web, USENET, and electronic mailing lists. This book does not explain how to use these applications. For general information about the Internet and guidance on how to use it, we suggest that you read the *1999 Canadian Internet New User's Handbook* or the *1999 Canadian Internet Handbook*.

Most chapters in this book make reference to various Web sites, and we have summarized Web site addresses at the end of the chapters. Since many Web sites change the locations of their individual pages on a frequent basis, we have avoided listing exact page references in this book. Instead, the Web site summaries at the end of the chapters will usually provide the main site addresses only.

We have made every effort to ensure that the Internet addresses contained in this book are accurate. All of the addresses were verified at the time of editing. But because the Internet is constantly changing, inevitably some resources will have changed their location or just disappeared. If you find an address that doesn't work, please let us know about it by sending an e-mail to **authors@handbook.com**. We will update the entry in subsequent editions of this book.

ACKNOWLEDGMENTS

We would like to thank the entire editorial, sales, marketing, and production team at Prentice Hall Canada for their effort on this book.

A special thanks to Robert Harris for skillfully and professionally managing all of our book projects. We would also like to acknowledge Judy Bunting and Joan Whitman on the editorial side; Andrea Aris, Michael Bubna, Trina Milnes, and Linda Voticky for their sales and marketing support; and Jan Coughtrey, Avivah Wargon, David Jolliffe, and Erich Volk for their production assistance.

To Betty Robinson, our editor: once again, thanks for your support and efforts on yet another book project.

We are grateful to i*STAR Internet, PSINet, Internet Light and Power, Rogers WAVE, Sympatico, and NETCOM Canada for the provision of Internet accounts and Web hosting services.

We also owe a big thanks to our families. Rick would like to thank his family for their continuing support. Jim would like to thank Christa, who went above and beyond the call of duty with this particular project.

A note of dedication to Jim's mom, an amazing woman who passed away while this book was in progress. She was so proud of her son and taught so many people about the joy to be found in the simple things in life.

Finally, we appreciate the ongoing support of our readers and fans and the millions of Internet users across Canada. This book would not be possible without you!

ABOUT THE AUTHORS

Jim Carroll, CA, is an internationally recognized Internet expert, popular media authority, and business consultant. He is author of the critically acclaimed book *Surviving the Information Age*, a motivational work that encourages people to cope with the future, and is a popular contributor to many leading Canadian publications. He has been recognized by *The Financial Post* as one of Canada's leading keynote speakers, providing motivating and challenging presentations for tens of thousands of North Americans at annual conferences, meetings, corporate events, and seminars. Clients include the Business Development Bank of Canada, the American Marketing Association, the Canadian Life and Health Assurance Association, the National Association of Fleet Administrators, Nortel, IBM, Remax, the Canadian Institute of Mortgage Brokers and Lenders, the CIBC, Montreal Trust, Great West Life, Scotia McLeod, the Royal Bank of Canada, Canada Trust, and many others. With his consulting practice, Mr. Carroll is noted for his ability to help organizations think strategically about the opportunity afforded by the Internet. Mr. Carroll is represented by several speakers bureaus worldwide that represent many of Canada's and the world's most widely recognized and popular political, entertainment, business, and technology personalities. He can be reached online by e-mail at **jcarroll@jimcarroll.com** or through his Web site, **www.jimcarroll.com**.

About the Authors

Rick Broadhead, MBA, is one of Canada's foremost Internet experts, industry observers, and a leading consultant and commentator on the Internet and the fast-growing field of electronic commerce. Mr. Broadhead has been retained as a keynote speaker, workshop facilitator, and consultant by businesses and associations across North America to help them understand how the latest electronic commerce trends will affect their industries. Rick also teaches at York University's Division of Executive Development in Toronto, where he has advised managers and senior executives from hundreds of leading North American firms and helped them integrate the Internet into all facets of their businesses. In his consulting practice, Mr. Broadhead assists organizations in formulating and implementing their Internet strategies. His expertise has been sought by Fortune 500 firms and many Canadian and North American industry leaders, including McDonald's, Microsoft Corporation, the Royal Bank of Canada, Sprint, VISA International, Imperial Oil, PolyGram, EMI Music, Manulife Financial, and Mackenzie Financial Services. He can be reached by e-mail at **rickb@sympatico.ca**, or visit his World Wide Web site at **www.rickbroadhead.com**.

YOUR EXPERIENCES WITH ONLINE FINANCE

We are always interested in hearing from our readers. We welcome your comments, criticisms, and suggestions and we will use your feedback to improve future editions of this book. We do try to respond to all e-mail sent to us.

We are also very interested in tracking how Canadians are using the Internet to manage their personal finances. How has the Internet helped you with your retirement or financial planning activities? Have you been a victim of online fraud? What financial resources do you find most helpful? What's your favourite investment site on the Web? If you'd like to share your online experiences with us, we'd love to hear from you. We might use your story in a future case study. Similarly, if you are aware of any Canadian organizations that are developing financial products or services for the online marketplace, please let us know so that we can make mention of them in future editions of this book.

Contacting the Authors Directly

To reach	Send e-mail to
Both authors	authors@handbook.com
Jim Carroll	jcarroll@jimcarroll.com
Rick Broadhead	rickb@sympatico.ca

Automatic E-mail Information

You can easily obtain current information about this book or any of our other books by sending a message to **info@handbook.com**. You will be sent back a message that will provide details on our books, our online resources, ordering instructions, and other relevant information.

Our World Wide Web Sites

The World Wide Web site for all our books is **www.handbook.com**. There you will find information about all of our publications, including press releases, reviews from the media, and ordering instructions.

Jim Carroll maintains a World Wide Web site at **www.jimcarroll.com**. He posts to this site, on a regular basis, articles that he has written about the Internet and the "information superhighway," including those from his weekly "e-biz" column in the *Globe and Mail*, as well as articles he has written for *Computing Canada*, the *Toronto Star, EnRoute, Strategy Magazine,* and other publications. The site also includes details about his speaking engagements, extensive video related to his work, and other background information about his activities.

Rick Broadhead maintains a World Wide Web site at **www.rickbroadhead.com**, with information about his work, his clients, and pointers to World Wide Web sites from his presentations and speeches about the Internet and the online world.

CHAPTER 1

Investing on the Internet

Twenty years from now you will be more disappointed by the things you didn't do than by the ones you did do. MARK TWAIN

HIGHLIGHTS

- Many Canadians recognize that they need to take on more responsibility for planning for their financial security during retirement. At the same time, they recognize that they need to improve their knowledge of investment matters.

- The Internet provides Canadians with an unprecedented amount of information on RRSPs, retirement planning, and investments in general. By accessing and using this information, Canadians can take more control over their own financial affairs.

- This book can be used by individuals comfortable with retirement and investment issues. If you are not, the four appendixes at the back will teach you about the basic retirement and investment issues, as well as describe how you can use the Internet to learn more about these topics.

The emergence of the Internet has contributed to a significant and important trend: many people are starting to take more responsibility for their own investment decisions. That is what this book is all about.

Will the Internet make you an expert when it comes to financial matters?

No, but it will certainly help you with some of the most important financial issues that you are faced with. It can help you develop a greater understanding of why you should be planning for your retirement today instead of putting it off to the future. Used wisely, the Internet can also help you make intelligent RRSP and other investment decisions.

> **For some time, Carlson On-line (www.carlsononline. com) has been tracking the number of Canadian public companies that have Web sites. By October 1998, over 2,000 Canadian public companies had their own Web sites. This compares to 150 in May 1996, 840 in May 1997, 1,200 in August 1997, and 1,600 in January 1998.**

The Internet can help to demystify what for many people is a mystery: the world of finance. The extent of investment and financial information on the Internet is truly amazing: the Internet represents the world's largest collection of financial information from all over the globe.

Here are some of the things that you can learn if you spend some time online:

- You can get a better understanding of what RRSPs are all about and why they are such an important financial tool.

- You can find out how much you need to save for your retirement and discover if you will have enough for your retirement, based on your current and future RRSP contributions.

- You can find out how much tax you can save with your current RRSP contributions.

- You can learn more about investing and discover how to use the Internet to determine what you should be investing in.

- You can quickly find out which financial institutions offer the best rates on term deposits and similar investments, or you can research the risk associated with the new cash-based investment products that so many financial organizations are offering.

CHAPTER 1: Investing on the Internet

- You can examine details of hundreds of mutual funds to help you decide which investments are best for you.
- You can quickly find the top-performing mutual funds in various investment categories.
- You can browse through an unprecedented range of information about the stock market and research tens of thousands of companies that you might invest in.
- You can buy and sell mutual funds and stocks online and save on commission fees.
- You can monitor the performance of your investments on a day-to-day basis so that you can see how your investments are working for you.

Regardless of your financial situation, you will discover the Internet to be an extremely effective and powerful financial tool.

> **Need statistics on investing in Canada? One of the best places to search is the Statistics Canada Web site (www.statcan.ca), which contains a wealth of information. Choose The Daily—a daily report of statistics being released—then choose to do an archive search.**

Survey After Survey...

As a financial tool, the Internet couldn't have come at a better time. Open any newspaper or magazine and you will find surveys that show most Canadians agree with two fundamental statements:

- They are concerned that they will have to take on more responsibility for their retirement, since they don't expect there to be enough money in government and private pension plans to take care of them.
- They need to learn more about RRSPs and retirement and investment issues.

Consider a study that was prepared for Scotiabank by the research firm Goldfarb Consultants in December 1996. The study found that:

- Canadians who are 45 and older estimate that 40% of their retirement income will have to come from personal savings and investments.

- 58% of Canadians have money set aside in an RRSP.

- While half of Canadians expressed a personal interest in investment matters, only two in ten felt they had an expert or high level of investment knowledge.

The bottom line? Canadians need to do a better job at managing their RRSP and investment activities, but they feel they don't have the knowledge to do so.

That's where the Internet comes in. Never before has there been a tool like the Internet that makes it possible for the average Canadian to effectively deal with these two pressing issues.

Mastering the Internet is a significant and often frustrating challenge for many people. Many feel overwhelmed by the amount of information online and are fearful about the possibility of being victimized by an online con artist.

> **Typically, I got my best ideas on where to look for investment information and trading Web sites from articles and reviews in newspapers and magazines—a sad if inevitable state of affairs for a medium that promises to solve all your information problems.**
>
> EDWARD H. BAKER, "ROUNDUP, INTERNET STYLE," *FINANCIAL WORLD*, JANUARY 21, 1997

We have written this book to help you learn how to use the Internet as an investment and retirement planning tool. You can use this book to learn:

- about fundamental retirement, RRSP, mutual fund, and investment issues;

- how to apply the Internet to your investment and retirement planning needs.

This book is designed for two groups of people:

- those who want a better understanding of issues related to investing in RRSPs; and

- those who want to learn more about investing online, both for general investment purposes and for purposes of retirement.

If you are in the second category, we suggest that you start out with appendixes A to D: "Learning About the Basics of Retirement Planning and RRSPs on the Internet," "Basic Investment Concepts," "Mutual Fund Concepts," and "Learning About Investments on the Internet." Reading these appendixes will be a useful primer not only on basic retirement and investment issues, but also on how you can use the Internet as a financial learning tool.

Throughout this book we provide plenty of examples that you can use to harness the power of the Internet when it comes to your own RRSP, retirement, mutual fund, and investment decisions. Mastering these capabilities is important. We sincerely believe that you will see dramatic payoffs if you take the time and effort to learn to effectively use the Internet.

Here's a guide to what you will find in the chapters that follow:

- In chapter 2, "The Benefits and Risks of Using the Internet for Online Investing," we explain the benefits of using the Internet as an investment and retirement planning aid, but also take a look at the dangers of using the Internet as a financial resource. We also describe how to be an "information skeptic" when it comes to information online.

- In chapter 3, "Determining What to Invest In," we discuss the types of decisions you will face as you decide where to invest your money.

- In chapter 4, "Using Financial Calculators," we describe how you can use interactive calculators on the Internet to appreciate the time value of money. Use these calculators, and we are certain that you will be propelled into action!

- In chapter 5, "Cash and Cash-Equivalent Investments on the Internet," we explain how the Internet can help you research cash-based and cash-equivalent offerings from financial institutions. These investments include savings accounts, Canada Savings Bonds, guaranteed investment certificates, and term deposits.

- In chapter 6, "Mutual Funds on the Internet," we describe some of the tools that you can use to research mutual funds on the Internet.

- In chapter 7, "Researching Stocks and Bonds on the Internet," we outline how you can use the Internet to research existing or potential investments in stocks and bonds and how to perform company and market research online.

- In chapter 8, "Online Investing," we describe how you can use the Internet to buy and sell mutual funds, stocks, bonds, and other financial instruments.

- In chapter 9, "Monitoring Your Performance," we show you how you can use powerful tools on the Internet to track the value and performance of your investments on a day-to-day basis.

- Finally, in chapter 10, "Don't Become Overconfident," we examine what we think are some of the key concerns for those seeking to empower themselves as investors on the Internet.

You Do Not Have to Be a Brilliant Computer Geek to Read This Book

This book has been written with the assumption that readers have a working knowledge of the Internet. This book does not describe the fundamentals of sending e-mail and using the World Wide Web. Rather, it describes how you can apply the Internet to your financial needs.

For an introduction to the Internet, how it works, and how to use basic Internet tools like e-mail and the Web, we recommend that you consult the *Canadian Internet New User's Handbook*.

Let's move on!

CHAPTER 2

The Benefits and Risks of Using the Internet for Online Investing

If a million people believe a foolish thing, it is still a foolish thing. ANATOLE FRANCE

HIGHLIGHTS

- The Internet can save you money, keep you up-to-date, expose you to different perspectives on financial matters, and make the whole process of managing your investments a lot more enjoyable. Perhaps most importantly, the Internet is a vital tool that will empower you and give you a competitive edge in the marketplace.

- The Internet is the perfect environment for fraud artists: they can publish any information they want, create their own identities, and reach millions of people with little effort.

- Fraud on the Internet generally falls into one of the following four categories: manipulation of obscure, thinly traded stocks, unlicensed investment advisors, conflicts of interest, and exotic scams.

> - **Fraud can originate from several sources on the Internet, including electronic investment newsletters and Web sites, spam, newsgroups and chat sites, and bogus Web sites.**
> - **Investment information on the Internet can be inaccurate, out-of-date, and/or misleading. In addition, the information you come across may not be applicable to Canada.**
> - **It's important to learn to question the validity and credibility of any investment information that you access on the Internet.**
> - **Always check the credentials of the people you are dealing with online; use caution when taking investment advice from strangers, anonymous individuals, and people who claim to have inside information; don't buy thinly traded stocks on the basis of hype; and be aware that people may be getting paid to promote a stock on the Internet.**

We are convinced that the Internet is leading to a new era of empowerment for Canadian investors, because it so easily allows us to take on more responsibility for our RRSP, retirement, and investment decisions.

And that's what this book is all about. It provides guidance on how to master the Internet in these important areas.

Having said that, we must make two extremely important observations:

- The Internet is leading a lot of people to think they can "do it all on their own" when it comes to their investment activities, an issue that carries with it a certain degree of risk. We examine this issue in chapter 10, "Don't Become Overconfident."

- The Internet is full of fraudulent, misleading, and downright dishonest investment information.

In this chapter we take a look at the benefits that can come from using the Internet, but we also consider the risks that go along with it. Finally, we outline what you can do to protect yourself should you decide to use it as a retirement and investment tool.

The Benefits of Using the Internet for Your Retirement and Investment Decisions

Clearly, many people have come to discover the power of the Internet when it comes to retirement and investment decisions. After all, consider what it can provide:

1. Useful New Skills

There is no doubt that the Internet is here to stay and that it will forever change the world of finance.

Learning to research the Internet effectively and to take advantage of the information you find online is becoming increasingly important. It is particularly important when it comes to financial decisions concerning your investments, whether they be for your retirement or for other personal or business reasons.

2. Cost Savings

Once you are hooked up to the network, you can access most information on the Internet for free.

This makes the Internet an unprecedented research tool, providing access to very detailed and often "up-to-the-minute" financial information, all for an extremely reasonable cost. With Internet access in most major Canadian cities approaching a flat monthly fee of about $20 (a little more in rural areas), it is probably the most significant information bargain on the planet.

In addition, if you take on more responsibility for your financial affairs, you can save significant sums of money. For example, if you learn how to undertake your own stock trades on a service such as E*Trade Canada, you can save money on stockbroker commissions. You can also use the Internet to find the best no-load or commission-free mutual funds instead of going with "load" funds that involve a commission paid to the financial professional who sells them to you.

These are but two examples of the direct savings that the Internet can help you to achieve.

> **Competition in the online brokerage industry in the United States in 1998 led to substantial cuts in commission fees, in some cases as low as $9.95.**

3. Motivation

Investment and retirement decisions can be, for many people, quite boring.

But the Internet can turn complex, laborious, or even boring financial tasks into a stimulating experience. Many people find that when they plug into the Internet, their perspective on the world of finance changes. Suddenly, financial matters seem more interesting and more manageable. The Internet can generate enthusiasm for routine tasks, thereby giving people an added incentive to deal with their financial affairs.

4. Responsibility

Learn about some of the issues we outline in this book, and then visit the sites we recommend. After studying the information, we are willing to bet that your attitude toward certain financial issues will change forever.

We think that once you learn to take advantage of the rich financial information that the Internet offers, you will begin to use it more and, as a result, become more aggressively involved in your own financial affairs. Which is a good thing, since study after study show two consistent trends in Canada: Canadians feel in the dark when it comes to retirement and financial issues, and they want to become more involved in these areas.

5. Power

The Internet is slowly tipping the scales of many financial relationships in your favour, since it is helping to introduce new forms of competition into the financial services industry. It helps you, the consumer, by giving you more power.

In the world of finance this is significant. You can now make quick comparisons between investment or savings rates at different banks, trust companies, and credit unions; undertake a quick analysis to find the best-performing mutual funds in a specific category or research the background of various mutual funds so that you can determine which works best for you; and learn more about new financial offerings from banks and other companies to educate yourself about the risks that they don't mention in their advertisements.

The Internet empowers you because you no longer have to rely solely on the information provided by stockbrokers or other investment advisors.

In effect, you can become a more informed investor. And you will likely experience a new feeling of satisfaction by mastering your own financial affairs.

6. Timeliness

One of the most powerful aspects of the Internet is that you can use it to keep up-to-date on your investments and keep abreast of changes in government policy that might affect your financial position upon retirement.

Think about this: today you might receive or obtain pamphlets and brochures from financial organizations or read about various financial alternatives in the newspaper. But due to the rapid rate of change in the world of finance, you will often discover that such information is out-of-date as soon as it is printed.

The world of finance changes on an almost daily basis, making it a challenge to obtain up-to-date information when you need it. And the complexity of the world means that you can't afford to be *unaware* of how you might be impacted by changes in the financial industry.

This is where the Internet comes in. Many Web sites contain the latest, most up-to-date, and most accurate information available, which will enable you to make more informed financial decisions.

Never before has it been so easy for investors to keep themselves current on financial matters, whether interest rates, stock prices, investment or business news, or political developments around the world. And with the emergence of online "portfolio tools," you can even track the day-to-day value of your investments.

7. A Global Perspective

Face it—many Canadians tend to get too focused on issues like national unity and the deficit and on hockey.

But plug into the Internet, and you suddenly acquire an international perspective. You can now access opinions and expertise from financial professionals all over the world. Access to the world stage can influence your investment and other financial decisions.

> "Doing business on the Internet is 'orders of magnitude' less expensive compared with providing more traditional services such as toll-free telephone numbers and customer support representatives," said George G. Hathaway, III, vice president of strategic planning for Fidelity's retail group.
>
> JOHANNA AMBROSIO, "FIDELITY POSTS 'NET SERVICES,'" *COMPUTERWORLD*, AUGUST 25, 1997

8. Different Perspectives

There are many different approaches when dealing with investment matters. Journey onto the Internet and you will discover that it provides all kinds of different viewpoints and ideas, each of which you can carefully evaluate when making financial decisions. You will learn to appreciate the dictum that there is no right answer.

9. A Full Range of Financial Information

The more financial organizations that get involved with the Internet and establish Web sites, the more information-rich you become.

The quantity—and quality—of information on the Internet is stunning. Since the World Wide Web burst onto the scene in early 1993, the Internet has become the largest depository of financial information on the planet. It provides instant access to information on retirement planning, RRSPs, mutual funds, stocks, bonds, GICs, and almost every other conceivable investment topic.

The Risks of Using the Internet as an Investment Tool

Even though the Internet can be a powerful companion for your investment and retirement decisions, we also believe that it presents the investor with *significant* risk, unless you take care with its use.

The fact is that there is a tremendous opportunity for you to make bad, invalid, or incorrect retirement and investment decisions based on the information you might find online. The Internet is proving to be fertile ground for online fraud, misinformation, and rumour. Not only that, but the information you rely on could be wrong—simply out-of-date or incorrect. And finally, the Internet is not a panacea: while it is a wonderful tool to assist the investment decision-making process, it is but one facet of what you need to properly manage your investments.

Hence, before we begin to examine specific retirement and investment issues in this book, we feel we *must* first put into perspective the risks of using the Internet as an information tool and provide some guidance on how you can evaluate the credibility of the information you find online.

Many of our comments in this chapter have to do with investment fraud involving stocks. This is because the stock market is subject to a greater degree of risk and manipulation than other financial industries. While fraud certainly does occur in other financial industries, it is less common than stock fraud. Even so, the guidance in this chapter is applicable to any investment information that you might access on the Internet.

Why Do Scam Artists Love the Internet?

If a fraud artist had been asked a couple of years ago to dream up the perfect tool to commit investment fraud, he or she probably would not have been able to come up with anything as perfect as the Internet. The Internet is made for the fraud artist; it's almost too good to be true.

Why? Because it is very easy to create your own identity on the Internet, one that has absolutely nothing to do with the truth. And because many people are gullible: all too many people believe what they read online, without taking the time to judge the validity of the information they are accessing.

> **Use common sense. Ask yourself, If this investment is so enticing, why am I being selected for this great opportunity? Common sense is your best protection against fraud.**
> GRETCHEN MORGENSOM, "DON'T BE A VICTIM," *FORBES*, JUNE 2, 1997, V159 N11 PP:42-43

Online Fraud 101

It is easy enough to use the Internet to take advantage of people. If we wanted to, we could create an elaborate scheme that recommends investing in a certain company that makes peanut butter. The basis of our scheme would be this: we would announce that, because scientists have just figured out that an ingredient in this particular brand of peanut butter has been shown to result in a dramatic decrease in colon cancer, investment in this company is a good bet.

How would we go about pulling this off? First of all, we would create a report from a fictitious "independent" research institute, distribute it to a few key health groups online, and invite people to visit our Web site to learn more. This would help to get a buzz going in some health areas on the Internet. Sadly, a lot of people access medical information on the Internet without questioning its accuracy, a topic we explore in our book *Good Health Online—A Wellness Guide for Every Canadian*.

We would create this Web site in a way that clearly authenticated our claims. We would create enthusiastic—but bogus—reports from the medical community as well as fictitious news articles. We would have a series of press releases describing the research that had been reported worldwide about the link between this particular ingredient in peanut butter and colon cancer.

We would also hit a few online investment discussion forums and create numerous identities for ourselves. These identities would be used to create an entirely phony "discussion" between three or four "different" people debating the research results. We would even create an identity for a medical doctor who would join the online discussions and comment enthusiastically about the product.

We would pay a few more people to make their own enthusiastic postings online, recognizing that there are individuals out there who will do this for a fee.

We would try to stimulate the interest of online investment newsletters to help publicize our findings.

We would target, through e-mail, investors whose e-mail addresses we found through online discussion forums. We would send them highly enthusiastic reports that "this investment is a sure bet!" and that "you can't lose on this one!" We would appeal to that most base of human emotions, greed.

And of course, behind the scenes, we would have purchased shares in the company and would plan to sell them once the price rose and make some easy money in the process.

Far-fetched? Sadly, no. It happens much too frequently on the Internet.

The Perfect Environment for Fraud

Why is the Internet such a popular target for scam artists? Consider what the Internet provides:

- **The world's largest printing press**

  Anyone can publish information about anything on the Internet. And as has been reported over and over, the Internet is difficult, if not impossible, to regulate. This means that it's easy for scam artists to spread inaccurate and fraudulent information to an audience of millions of people.

- **A lack of information skepticism**

  The sad reality is that if we did create the peanut butter story we described above, some people out there would believe it. We are stunned that people are so gullible.

  There are a lot of people on the Internet who are too willing to believe what they read online without subjecting the information to an adequate degree of what we call "information skepticism."

> In an article entitled "Don't Be a Victim" in the June 2, 1997, issue of *Forbes*, the chief of enforcement of the Securities and Exchange Commission (SEC) spoke about Comparator Systems, a company that the SEC shut down for fraudulent activity in 1995. The SEC chief noted that the Internet was primarily responsible for "much of the investment" in Comparator Systems, since all kinds of investors were purchasing the stock based on "hot Internet tips" about the company.

These people are lulled into a false sense of security when it comes to information on the Internet. This makes the Net a particularly dangerous tool when it comes to the world of investing, because many scam artists recognize this fact and target investment chat sites such as that found on Silicon Investor on the Internet.

- **A new identity**

  It's easy for people to conceal their true identities on the Internet. In fact, you can be anyone you like and therefore say anything you like with very little fear of repercussions. This situation will last until regulatory authorities figure out how to deal with the Internet, if they can.

  Consider the following. There are a lot of free e-mail services on the Internet that you can sign up with. We went to one, applied for an e-mail address with a user-ID of "Jean Chretien," and received it within a matter of minutes. We were able to send e-mail to friends and relatives with a return e-mail address that made the messages appear as though they were coming from someone named Jean Chretien.

  Next, we assumed the personas of John Felderhof and Bill Gates. We could have easily posted a few messages to investment discussion forums under their names.

  Is this legal? Probably not. Is it ethical? Certainly not. Is it easy to do? Most definitely. It is very easy to become whomever you want to be online.

  As an investor looking for information online, you have absolutely no assurance of the identity of the people or organizations with whom you might communicate on the Internet.

  In addition to forging e-mail addresses and assuming a false identity in a chat group, fraud artists have been known to set up bogus Web sites that impersonate official Web sites.

- **Massive reach**

  The Internet presents the scam artist with a global audience and the ability to reach millions of people with minimal effort. Never before has there been a technology that makes it so easy for so few to defraud so many.

- **A technology that is difficult to regulate**
  Scam artists love the Internet because it's so difficult to police. Government and legal authorities as well as securities regulators are having a tough time curtailing investment fraud on the Internet.

  Consider what was said by the North American Securities Administrators Association (NASAA), which bills itself as "the oldest international organization devoted to investor protection": "Even if the several thousand people in the United States who work at the Securities and Exchange Commission (SEC), state securities agencies, National Association of Securities Dealers (NASD), and the stock exchanges were somehow able to put aside all other tasks in a massive bid to shut down online investment scams, it is doubtful that this problem could be stamped out altogether."

- **Ease of execution**
  Finally, scams are easy to perpetrate. Think about the peanut butter scam we described above. It would be very easy for us to expand upon those thoughts and write a step-by-step book called "How to Conduct an Effective Investment Fraud on the Internet."

  It wouldn't be a difficult book to write; we could describe the techniques in just a few short pages. Sad to say, it would probably be a bestseller.

  We're joking of course, but we are also quite serious about the prevalence of fraud—it is very easy for *anyone* to come up with an effective Internet investment scam. That is perhaps the scariest thing about the Internet when it comes to the world of finance.

Considering the facts we've enumerated above, it's important to develop a good sense of information skepticism as you use the Internet for investment purposes. For more on this, see the section "Evaluating the Credibility and Validity of Online Information" later in this chapter.

Types of Online Fraud

In addition to understanding why fraud is so easy to perpetrate on the Internet, it's important that you become familiar with the different ways that an online fraud can occur.

NASAA has identified the four most common types of fraud that occur on the Internet: manipulation of obscure, thinly traded stocks, unlicensed investment advisors, conflicts of interest, and exotic scams.

Manipulation of Obscure, Thinly Traded Stocks

Many of the most common investment scams involve small, relatively unknown stocks that aren't traded very frequently. These are called "thinly traded stocks" because they aren't traded very often. Some fraud artists attempt to inflate the value of little-known stocks, taking advantage of their low profile to make a quick profit.

They do this by making claims about "awesome new discoveries" or "significant new developments" relating to these companies. This often results in a flurry of buying activity, which in turn raises the stock price. As the stock price rises, others begin to take notice of the company, causing even more stock purchases and an even higher stock price. A buying frenzy begins with a sudden and sharp increase in the stock price. Everyone wants in!

Fraud artists profit from this type of activity by buying their shares at a low price and then cashing them in once the stock price reaches a certain level. Everyone else is left holding the bag, losing money when the price of the stock eventually collapses upon discovery of the bogus information.

Unlicensed Investment Advisors

In North America, you must be licensed by an appropriate provincial, territorial, or state authority in order to provide advice on the buying or selling of securities. In Canada, provincial and territorial securities commissions regulate the licensing of investment advisors. Many of the people who offer investment advice on the Internet aren't qualified to be dispensing such advice, and they are doing so illegally because they aren't licensed.

The Ontario Securities Commission (OSC) is aware of the problem. In 1997 they shut down a Web site called the Federal Bureau of Investments because the person operating the site was offering investment advice without being registered with the Commission.

But think about this: the Internet doesn't know about provincial or national borders. How does the OSC deal with someone based in Utah offering advice about a Canadian stock?

Conflicts of Interest

It is common practice for companies to pay promoters to hype their stocks on the Internet. The fact that the promoters are being paid to say positive things about the company and its stock is often not disclosed to investors who are reading the information.

For example, in 1997 a Florida stock promoter by the name of George Chelekis was charged by the U.S. Securities and Exchange Commission after it was discovered that he had accepted at least $1.1 million from more than 150 companies, as well as 275,500 shares of stock from 10 companies, in exchange for recommending their stock on his Web site. Chelekis, who distributed a newsletter on the Internet called "Hot Stocks Review," was charged by the Commission for "materially false and misleading statements" concerning six publicly traded companies as well as for failing to disclose the fact that he was receiving money from the companies he was promoting.

Think about what can happen on the Internet. Someone establishes an online newsletter full of investment tips and advice. But behind the scenes, the person writing the publication is receiving money from the very companies that he promotes in his newsletter.

Exotic Scams

Exotic scams are schemes where investors are promised big returns in exchange for making large investments in a venture.

A popular type of exotic scam is the pyramid scheme. Typical pyramid schemes sign up people to be distributors for certain products and/or services and then promise to pay those people commissions if they recruit even more distributors.

You should be cautious of any venture that claims you will make money by recruiting new members instead of by selling products or services yourself.

How serious is this problem? In just *one day* of searching the Web in late 1996, the U.S. Federal Trade Commission and other law enforcement agencies found over

500 Web sites that may have been involved in illegal pyramid schemes. Don't fall for these scams.

Common Sources of Online Fraud

Having discussed the most popular types of online fraud, you may be wondering where fraud is most likely to occur on the Internet. There are four primary sources: electronic newsletters and Web sites, spam, newsgroups and chat sites, and bogus Web sites.

Electronic Newsletters and Web Sites

There are countless numbers of investment newsletters on the Internet and massive numbers of investment-oriented Web sites. Any one of these could be a scam. As we pointed out earlier, anyone can publish on the Internet.

> **Janice Shell has become somewhat famous in the Internet investment community and has earned the title cyber-vigilante. A fifty-year-old art historian living in Milan, she spends about twelve hours a day on the Internet seeking out and exposing con men and false Web sites. To demonstrate how easy it is to fool people online, she created an elaborate Web site about a fake company, FBN Associations (FBN stands for Fly By Night) and began to publicize it in various online investment forums. How gullible are people? She even included a press release within the corporate Web site that the company received a papal blessing. Even that stretch of the imagination did not turn people away—she was inundated with messages from people asking how they could invest in the company.**

Spam

If you have an Internet e-mail address, you have no doubt received electronic junk mail, which is often referred to as "spam" or "junk e-mail."

An increasing number of junk e-mail messages promote investment opportunities, many of them fraudulent. Fraud artists are discovering that they can use the Internet to send a message to millions of people for a very low cost. Inevitably, they will draw some people in.

Newsgroups and Chat Sites

If you want to see how the Internet can influence what people do with their investments, spend some time browsing an Internet newsgroup (discussion group) or an investment chat site such as Silicon Investor.

In their StockTalk section you can join any number of discussion areas about particular stocks and companies. Read some of the messages in the forums, and you'll see all kinds of claims about the future of certain stocks.

As you read this information, keep in mind the risks that we described earlier. How do you know that any of these people are real investors? How do you know that these participants making enthusiastic comments about specific stocks aren't being paid to do so? How do you know that two people posting messages under different identities aren't really the same person?

Online discussion forums can be useful and powerful tools, but they are also one of the primary methods used by scam artists. To use them effectively, you must have a level head and a very strong sense of information skepticism. Otherwise, you are the perfect target for a scam artist. Be vigilant at all times.

Bogus Web Sites

Finally, the Securities and Investments Board in the United Kingdom has warned that "copycat" Web sites are being set up by "unscrupulous operators who copy the Web pages of legitimate firms and then set up bogus ones of their own, passing themselves off as the real thing."

In other words, fraud artists are creating forgeries of investment sites on the Internet, with the intent of tricking Internet users into thinking they're looking at the real thing. Scary indeed.

Other Online Risks

The risk of fraud isn't the only problem you should be conscious of as you use the Internet. Even information that is placed online by reputable, established organizations often suffers from problems that affect its reliability.

Many of the issues above are specific to stocks or might not occur as frequently with other types of investments as they do with stocks. But the issues that follow are applicable to any type of investment, including mutual funds.

1. The information you access might be incorrect.
Always keep this in mind: there is no guarantee that anything you read online is accurate or true. Mistakes happen. Consider what happened in the United Kingdom in mid-1997: following crucial talks between the finance minister and the governor of the Bank of England, Britain's Treasury Department reported on the Internet that the governor had asked for a half-point rise in interest rates, when in fact he had asked for a quarter-point rise. Fortunately, the error was quickly identified, but only after the incorrect news had reached Britain's financial markets.

2. Information might be out-of-date.
When accessing financial information on the Internet, you might rely on information that is out-of-date and, hence, technically incorrect.

Many organizations are still experimenting with the Internet and have yet to commit the necessary funds to ensure that their sites are kept up-to-date at all times.

When you visit a financial Web site on the Internet, always try to ascertain when the site was last updated. Sometimes Web sites don't provide this information, and it's difficult to tell if the information you are reading was created yesterday or twelve months ago. Needless to say, it's dangerous to rely on outdated information for the purpose of making important investment decisions.

3. Information might not be applicable to Canada.
And always try to ascertain what country the site is in. Why is this important? If you're accessing advice on a Web site that is based in the United States, the advice being offered might not be applicable to Canada. In addition, the products or services being advertised might not be available in this country.

The global nature of the Internet means that you could find yourself using irrelevant information—and making an incorrect decision as a result.

> The U.S. Securities and Exchange Commission, in discussing the problem of online fraud, reported one situation in which not only was a fake company Web site created, but an entirely false magazine was created. The publication, World Financial Report, provided a glowing article about the false company.

4. The online tools you rely on might be wrong.

In this book we recommend a number of online calculators that can help you with your investment decisions as well as assist you in understanding the financial implications of retirement.

Who is to say that such calculators are correct? How do you know they have been programmed properly? How do you know that they have been updated to reflect recent tax or interest rate changes? How do you know that the assumptions used in these calculators are valid for your particular financial circumstances?

The answer is: you don't.

5. The information might be misleading.

The Internet can purport to make complex financial decisions seem all too easy. For example, there are sites that we describe in this book that will help you "choose" what types of investments are appropriate for you. These sites simplify what are really complex decisions.

Avoid blind reliance on these Web sites; use the information they provide only as guidance.

6. Your privacy might be violated.

You should be aware that your personal privacy is at risk when you use the Internet.

For example, many Web sites ask you to register or answer a series of questions before you are allowed to access the information or tools the site makes available. The information you provide might be sold to a telemarketing/direct mail firm or added to a database without your consent or knowledge.

For example, in chapter 9 we describe how you can use an online mutual fund/stock tracking service at various sites belonging to the Southam newspaper group. What we do not discuss in that chapter is the fact that

Southam wants you to fill out a form and provide your name, income, net worth, occupation, and other personal information.

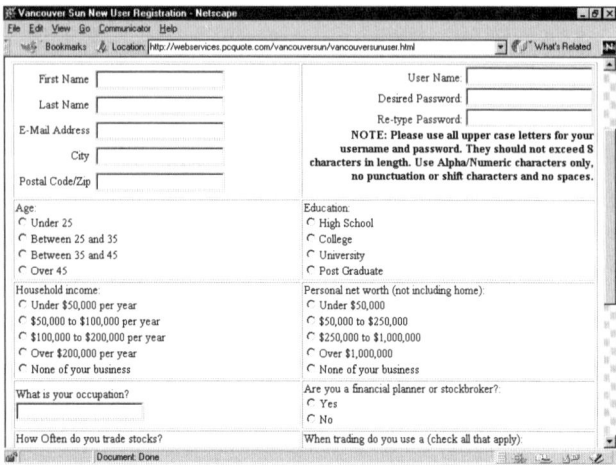

Now think about this: if you go ahead and fill out the form, there is no legislation in Canada (except in the province of Quebec) to prevent this company from doing whatever they like with the information that you've just willingly provided.

There are plenty of other examples on the Web. Recognizing that this practice worries a lot of Internet users, some companies have published privacy policies on their Web sites, which explain how they intend to use the information they collect from you.

What do we suggest? Always be careful in providing personal information online. If you don't have to provide it as part of a legally binding economic contract, then don't; in response to this type of information request, two-thirds of the people surveyed said they provide a pseudonym or other nonidentifying information.

7. You might experience technical problems.

Imagine this: you sign up for an online stock trading service and use it for a few months. Then one day, you need to sell the shares that you own in a particular company. You want to get rid of them urgently, since you are quite convinced that their price is going to drop dramatically.

You try to connect to the Internet, but you can't get through, and all you get is a busy signal. You keep trying and trying, and finally you manage to connect. Then you go to the Web site of your online trading service, only to find it intolerably slow. Finally, you get to the screen where you can sell your shares, and you begin entering the necessary details. Wham! Your Web browser crashes, you're disconnected from the Internet, and you get that nasty little "This Program Has Terminated Abnormally" message.

You redial your Internet provider, and you get a busy signal again...

By the time you manage to sell your shares, they've dropped 30% in price. Or to put it another way, the time you lost trying to connect to the online brokerage cost you an extra $3,000.

Is our story unrealistic? Not at all. Technical problems can occur at any time. In one widely reported case in the United States in 1997, a computer glitch at discount brokerage firm Charles Schwab meant that many of its customers were unable to determine whether their mutual fund and stock trades had been carried out.

The Bottom Line?

Have we scared you away? Do all these risks mean that you should shy away from using the Internet? Not at all. But always use caution when accessing investment information from this source. In particular, you should always question the *validity* and *credibility* of information you access online.

It's possible for information to be credible, but not valid. How so? When accessing investment information on the Internet, you need to consider factors such as the following:

- Is the information applicable to your own financial circumstances?

- Is the information applicable to Canada?

- Is the information accurate?

- Is the information up-to-date?

In other words, just because information comes from a credible source doesn't mean that it is accurate or applicable to your specific financial situation. There is a lot of outdated information on the Internet. By the same token, there is a lot of information on the Web that contains mistakes, even though it comes from highly respectable sources. Don't take anything you read on the Internet for granted. Before acting on any information that you received online, consult a financial advisor or other trusted professional or colleague.

A more serious problem on the Internet is the information that is neither credible nor valid. This type of information usually manifests itself in the form of a scam or fraud, which we discussed earlier.

Avoiding Fraud on the Internet

Regulatory authorities recognize that fraud is a serious problem on the Internet. Part of their response to the problem involves educating the public about the risks of obtaining investment advice off the Internet.

NASAA has published a document on its Web site called "Cyberspace Fraud and Abuse." It describes the most common methods for fraud to be perpetrated on the Internet. We highly recommend that you read it.

HOW A TYPICAL CYBER-SCHEME WORKS

"Is anyone out there following Company X?"

"I heard that Company X is about to make a major announcement. E-mail me or call this toll-free number to get an information package."

"I spoke to Company X's CEO, who confirmed details of next month's big news. I've bought 10,000 shares. Look for share price to double in the next month! Get it now!"

"Big news is just around the corner. We hear from a friend who has visited Company X that it is going to be even bigger than we thought. There's still time to get in."

"Short sellers are in the market! Keep the faith.... This will bounce back. The smart money will use the price as an opportunity to buy more and dollar average."

FROM THE NORTH AMERICAN SECURITY ADMINISTRATORS ASSOCIATION WEB SITE IN THE "INVESTOR EDUCATION" SECTION. "CYPERSPACE FRAUD AND ABUSE" (**www.nasaa.org**)

Here are some of the basic assumptions and attitudes that you should carry with you as you use the Internet for investment purposes.

10 Tips for Avoiding Fraud on the Internet

1. Don't expect to get rich quickly.
2. Question the validity of any information you read online.
3. Don't rely on securities regulators to police the Internet.
4. Don't buy thinly traded stocks on the basis of online hype.
5. Don't make any investment decisions based on the advice of someone who conceals his or her identity.
6. Don't trust strangers.
7. Treat any claims about "insider information" with suspicion.
8. Be aware that people may be getting paid to hype an investment.
9. Check the credentials of those you deal with.
10. There are rules to protect you.

1. Don't expect to get rich quickly.

If the information you find on the Internet sounds too good to be true, it probably is.

People have an amazing capacity to suspend their disbelief when it comes to money and investments, and they often end up doing something that they later regret. Don't let this happen to you.

Some of the claims that you will see on Web sites, in investment newsletters, and in discussion groups on the Internet are so obviously false it is hard to believe that people fall for the claims that are made. Suggestions that you can "double your money is six months," that an investment is a "guaranteed sure thing," or that "you, too, can share in the wealth explosion" should immediately set off alarm bells in your head.

Unbelievably, many people fall for such pitches. The fraud artists wouldn't be working the Internet as hard as they do if the public wasn't so easy to victimize. Fortunately, investor education programs such as those undertaken by the NASAA are helping to combat the problem.

2. Question the validity of any information you read online.

Earlier we talked about how you must develop a degree of information skepticism as you use the Internet.

If you plan on using the Internet to assist you with your financial decisions, it is important that you learn to judge the validity of what you read. This is such an important topic that we discuss it in more depth later in the chapter.

3. Don't rely on securities regulators to police the Internet.

Securities administrators, stock exchanges, financial institutions, governments, and the rest of the financial industry are still coming to grips with the problem of investment fraud on the Internet.

Some stock exchanges and provincial securities commissions do employ staff who monitor the Internet for illegal activity, but given the sheer size of the Internet, the fact that it's borderless, and the ease with which fraud artists can conceal their identities, these efforts aren't always successful.

Recognizing how massive the problem is, some regulatory bodies are looking for ways to automate surveillance on the Internet. In the United States, the National Association of Securities Dealers (NASD) has developed a program that will automatically search Web sites on the Internet for evidence of fraud.

However, many of these activities are in their early stages and are by no means comprehensive. You are very much on your own.

It's not easy being a financial regulator these days.
"CHALLENGES OF THE FINANCIAL CYBERCOP," *INSTITUTIONAL INVESTOR*, APRIL 1997, V31 N4 P:99

---

4. Don't buy thinly traded stocks on the basis of online hype.

Recall our discussion on thinly traded stocks in the section "Types of Online Fraud." On the Internet, outrageous claims are often made about these stocks, leading to a frenzy of trading activity and a sudden increase in the share price.

It is possible that such bursts of activity are legitimate, but they should make you suspicious. Our advice? Be cautious.

You should also be aware that certain stock exchanges have a less-than-savoury reputation and represent many of the thinly traded stocks that are often used for scams. For example, the Vancouver Stock Exchange (VSE) has been referred to in such publications as *Forbes* magazine as the scam capital of the world, and the Alberta Stock Exchange (ASE) has suffered from its share of problems with the manipulation of small, relatively unknown stocks.

Both exchanges indicate they are working hard to clean up their reputations, but there is no doubt that extra caution is in order when dealing with VSE- or ASE-listed stocks.

That's not to say that the other major Canadian exchanges in Montreal and Toronto have entirely clean reputations. The TSE, for example, has had its reputation battered and bruised by the Bre-X scandal.

5. Don't make any investment decisions based on the advice of someone who conceals his or her identity.

Why would you? How could you?

There are many places on the Internet where you can participate in online discussions about specific companies. Two of the most popular sites for investment discussions are The Motley Fool and Silicon Investor. Silicon Investor seems to be the most popular, with the company claiming that 70% of all online financial discussions take place on its Web site. Both of these sites allow users to remain anonymous and use other identities instead of their real names.

You need to exercise caution when obtaining investment information from any online discussion group. Even if a person reveals his true identity, how do you know he is who he says he is?

6. Don't trust strangers.

Not only should you not trust people who post information to the Internet under a false identity, but you should be wary of strangers in general.

Some people are very good at winning your confidence online. They will tell you that they have personally checked out an investment opportunity and that there is nothing you should be worried about.

Are you prepared to risk your hard-earned money on promises made by someone you don't even know?

Because it's difficult to judge the character of anyone you meet online, you need to be careful.

7. Treat any claims about "insider information" with suspicion.

If you browse investment discussion groups and financial Web sites, you'll find all kinds of people who purport to be "in the know." They say they know someone inside the company or someone in the industry or someone close to the boyfriend of the daughter of the CEO. They're "in the loop." Or so they say.

Always treat such claims with extreme suspicion.

8. Be aware that people may be getting paid to hype an investment.

Again, recall our discussion in "Types of Online Fraud" on conflicts of interest. It is sad but true that sometimes companies pay people to "talk up" their stock online—either on Web sites or in investment discussion forums. In most cases, the people doing the promoting do not disclose the fact that they're being paid to publicize the stock. These paid promoters sometimes pose as investors in investment discussion forums and plant positive rumours designed to drive up the price of a company's stock.

9. Check the credentials of those you deal with.

The law in Canada and the United States is clear: only registered securities dealers/investment advisors may provide advice regarding the purchase of securities. And they can only advise people in the province where they are registered. This means that someone who is registered with the British Columbia Securities Commission to sell stocks in British Columbia should not be advising people in Alberta. And someone who is registered with the Alberta Securities Commission (but not with the British Columbia Securities Commission) should not be advising residents of British Columbia. Of course, it is next to impossible to enforce these rules on the Internet.

Mutual funds can be sold by all kinds of groups, such as the sales force for mutual fund companies, banks, trust companies, as well as personal financial planners and brokers. These sales take place with little regulation. For several years the OSC has been trying to proclaim that it has the right to regulate the mutual funds industry in Ontario but has had no success to date. Hence, the industry is not regulated to the same extent as securities as described above. As a result, it is critical that you check out the qualifications and credibility of whomever you might be buying your mutual funds from.

On the Internet there is obviously a challenge with credibility—thousands of people provide investment advice and counsel on the Internet each and every day, by way of investment newsletters, Web sites, comments in discussion forums, electronic mail, and other electronic

TIPS ON NOT FALLING PREY TO A CON ARTIST

Avoiding being hurt by a con artist is as easy as doing your homework—before you invest.

Contact your provincial securities regulator...to see if the investment vehicle and the person selling it are registered.

Your provincial securities regulator will also be able to tell you if the salesperson has a disciplinary history; that is, whether any civil, criminal or administrative proceedings have been brought against him or her.

Contact your local Better Business Bureau to see if any complaints have been filed against the venture's promoters or principals.

Deal only with dealers or advisers having a proven track record.

Ask for written information on the investment product and the business. Such information, including financial data on the company and the risks involved in the investment, is contained in a prospectus. Read it carefully. Don't take everything you hear or read at face value. Ask questions if you don't understand, and do some sleuthing for yourself. If you need help in evaluating the investment, go to someone independent whom you can trust such as an attorney or an accountant.

Steer clear of investments touted with no down-side or risk.

FROM THE B.C. SECURITIES COMMISSION WEB SITE, IN THE SECTION "BE AN INFORMED INVESTOR" (**www.bcsc.bc.ca**)

means. Many people don't have the credentials to provide such advice and, hence, are providing it illegally.

Provincial securities commissions in Canada are beginning to crack down on unlicensed individuals who are dispensing investment advice on the Internet. For example, in 1997 the OSC shut down the Web site of one individual who was providing investment advice without being licensed. However, we can just imagine how many other individuals remain online, far beyond the reach of the OSC, in jurisdictions beyond the reach of Ontario and Canadian law.

If in doubt about someone's credentials, you should check with the appropriate securities regulator to find out if the person is licensed to provide advice on buying or selling securities. In Canada, this means checking with your provincial or territorial securities commission. In the United States, check with the state securities agency.

10. There are rules to protect you.

There are strict bylaws and regulations governing advertising by investment firms that are members of the Investment Dealers Association of Canada (IDA). The IDA is a self-regulating body within the Canadian securities industry that ensures that its members operate according to certain rules. IDA member firms and their employees who wish to advertise on the Internet must have their Web materials approved by a designated official within the firm who is responsible for advertising. Advertising must also meet other criteria. For example, it must not:

- contain any untrue statement or omission of a material fact

- be false or misleading

- contain an unjustified promise of results

- contain any opinion or forecast of future events that is not clearly labelled as such

- fail to fairly present the potential risks to the client

- use unrepresentative statistics to suggest unwarranted or exaggerated conclusions or fail to identify the material assumptions made in arriving at these conclusions.

Canada's stock exchanges also have their own bylaws and rules concerning promotional activities and disclosure of pertinent company information by their member firms.

These rules are designed to protect you, the investor, and it's important for you to know that they do extend to the Internet. For purposes of enforcement, most regulatory bodies treat the Internet just like any other advertising medium.

> ### BE ALERT FOR TELLTALE SIGNS OF ONLINE INVESTMENT FRAUD
>
> Be wary of promises of quick profits, offers to share "inside" information, and pressure to invest before you have an opportunity to investigate.
>
> Be careful of promoters who use "aliases." Pseudonyms are common online, and some salespeople will try to hide their true identity. Look for other promotions by the same person. Words like "guarantee," "high return," "limited offer," and "as safe as a C.D." may be a red flag. No financial investment is "risk-free," and a high rate of return means greater risk.
>
> Watch out for offshore scams and investment opportunities in other countries. When you send your money abroad, and something goes wrong, it's more difficult to find out what happened and to locate your money.
>
> FROM THE SECURITIES AND EXCHANGE COMMISSION WEB SITE IN THE "INVESTOR ASSISTANCE & COMPLAINTS" SECTION. "INVESTOR ALERTS" (**www.sec.gov/consumer/b-alert.htm**)

Evaluating the Credibility and Validity of Online Information

Earlier in the chapter we discussed the importance of assessing the credibility and validity of information you access on the Internet. Here are some tips to help you do this.

10 Steps for Evaluating the Credibility and Validity of Online Information

1. Does the person or organization who created the site have a reputable track record?
2. Do the site creators list their credentials?
3. Is the information on the site subject to some type of review process?
4. Does the information seem to be professionally maintained, or does it seem "thrown together"?
5. What is the nature of the information?
6. Does the information seem to be too good to be true?
7. Can you back up the information with other independent sources?
8. Is the site updated frequently?
9. Does the site seem to simply want your money?
10. Are independent news reports available about the initiative?

1. Does the person or organization who created the site have a reputable track record?

When travelling through the Web, keep in mind that Web sites are prepared by many different people and organizations. You need to think about whether you can trust information from certain sources. Understanding the source of the information will help you judge the credibility and validity of what you read online. For example, when looking at a Web site, it's important to determine whether the site is being funded or financed by a particular organization. If this is the case, this might mean that the information in the site is biased toward the products or services of the sponsoring firm.

More than likely, sites created by banks, credit unions, trust companies, mutual fund companies, newspapers, and others will be more credible than those established by a layperson who just has an interest in a specific investment topic.

Initiatives by major organizations such as GLOBEfund, from the *Globe and Mail*, and The Fund Library, both of which are well financed and quite serious, are generally more credible than those initiatives that are done on a shoestring budget by small, relatively unknown companies. And initiatives that have been endorsed or sanctioned by a professional association bear more credence than sites that are not.

All kinds of factors such as these must weigh into your assessment of the validity and credibility of the information you are reading.

That's not to say that a page of information prepared by an investment professional or small company will be unreliable or incorrect. There are many excellent, reputable sources of information from smaller, lesser-known organizations.

2. Do the site creators list their credentials?

You can sometimes judge the validity of the information on a site by examining the background of the individuals or organizations who have put the site together.

Browse through the site, and see if it includes details on the background of the site's creators. Determine if investment professionals have assisted in the preparation and review of materials on the site. Find out what type of review process information on the Web site is subject to.

You should clearly understand that in the investment industry there is a difference between those who are licensed to advise on securities and those who can provide general financial advice. This is a real source of confusion for novice investors. Provincial securities commissions do not regulate financial planners, bank employees, or mutual fund salespeople, but they do regulate brokers. This difference is really important when evaluating the credentials of people who provide information on the Internet.

Finally, be on the lookout for bogus credentials. Sometimes people will list qualifications that they don't really have.

3. Is the information on the site subject to some type of review process?

Sometimes you will find a site that not only clearly and unequivocally indicates the background of the people involved with the site, but also indicates that the information contained on it has been subject to some form of approval process. This information can be helpful when evaluating the credibility of financial information you find on the Internet.

Although not usually mentioned on Web sites, remember that any online advertising by investment firms that are members of the IDA must be approved by an official of the firm.

4. Does the information seem to be professionally maintained, or does it seem "thrown together"?

Sometimes a quick tour of a site can give you a gut feeling for the quality of the information that it contains.

If you browse a Web site and discover a lot of broken links, pages that don't work, and evidence that the site isn't being maintained properly, this should diminish your confidence in the information the site provides. The same holds true if the site is poorly organized, shows poor use of grammar, or has a lot of spelling mistakes—all the things that would generate in you a lack of confidence in the information found on the site. The quality of the site is often indicative of the quality of the information found there.

5. What is the nature of the information?

There is a big difference in the information supplied on the Web site of the Royal Bank of Canada and a posting made by an individual in an online discussion forum. And the Web site of the Montreal Stock Exchange provides more reliable information than you might find in a small investment newsletter that is e-mailed to everyone on a mailing list.

Hence, you should consider the nature of the information you are dealing with. Corporate information sites from established organizations would rank as more reliable than a newsletter put out by a small group of amateur investors, and a news report would bear more credence than a posting in a chat room.

6. Does the information seem too good to be true?

If so, it probably is.

7. Can you back up the information with other independent sources?

Information that you find online should always be verified with additional, independent sources that suggest the same thing.

Never, never, never take something for granted that you read online without confirming it with other sources.

How can you check out details about a particular company or person you read about online? There are many information sources—both online and offline—that you can consult. For example, you should check with an investment or financial professional, such as an investment advisor or accountant, before acting on information you retrieve off the Web. In addition, check the information you obtain online against what is being reported in newspapers, magazines, and on radio and television. Also check out company annual reports and prospectuses.

> ...the SEC's point man on the Internet is uncertain of how much longer traditional regulation can ride this whirlwind. "Is it moving so quickly, with so many different influences, that for the first time, you're in a qualitatively different ball game?" asks SEC commissioner Steven Wallman.
>
> "CHALLENGES OF THE FINANCIAL CYBERCOP," INSTITUTIONAL INVESTOR, APRIL 1997, V31 N4 P:99

8. Is the site updated frequently?

If you encounter a site that has not been updated for some time, you should probably be leery of using the information found there. After all, the world of finance changes regularly. How can you rely on information from a site where the owners don't take the time to ensure that the information they provide is kept up-to-date?

9. Does the site seem to simply want your money?

If you visit many sites you will inevitably come across some that want your credit card number as quickly as possible. Be suspicious of any sites that seem overly interested in your money.

10. Are independent news reports available about the initiative?

Finally, doing a search for news articles about a particular site, the site's creators, or on a specific investment topic may often reveal information that helps you determine the validity of the information you are reading online. Sites that have been reviewed positively in the media often feature copies of these articles on their sites. Articles from independent news sources can help judge whether the information sources you are using are credible.

Keep in mind that positive media reports don't guarantee that the information you are reading is credible or valid. But it is another item in your checklist that may help you decide on the overall reliability of an online information resource.

Where to Get Help

If you're suspicious about an online investment opportunity, you want to report a scam, or you simply want to verify whether someone is licensed to sell securities in your province or territory, contact your provincial or territorial securities commission. NASAA has a search engine on its site that you can use to find the mailing addresses and e-mail addresses of securities regulators across Canada and the United States.

If you're interested in reading more about how you can protect yourself against fraud on the Internet, and investment fraud in general, visit the NASAA Web site.

Web Sites Mentioned in This Chapter

British Columbia Securities Commission	www.bcsc.bc.ca
Charles Schwab	www.schwab.com
E*Trade Canada	www.canada.etrade.com
The Fund Library	www.fundlibrary.com
GLOBEfund	www.globefund.com
Montreal Stock Exchange	www.me.org
The Motley Fool	www.fool.com
National Association of Securities Dealers	www.nasd.com
North American Securities Administration Association (NASAA)	www.nasaa.org
Ontario Securities Commission	www.osc.gov.on.ca
Royal Bank	www.royalbank.com

Silicon Investor	www.techstocks.com
Southam	www.southam.com
Toronto Stock Exchange	www.tse.com
U.K. Financial Services Authority	www.sib.co.uk
U.S. Securities & Exchange Commission	www.sec.gov
Vancouver Stock Exchange	www.vse.ca

CHAPTER 3

Determining What to Invest In

No great discovery was ever made without a bold guess. ISAAC NEWTON

HIGHLIGHTS

- When it comes to investing, everyone has a theory. It is important to learn that no theory is definitive and there are no absolutely right answers.

- The best way to determine what to invest in is to educate yourself about the different categories and types of investments and think about how these investments relate to the characteristics of risk, growth, and income.

- You will encounter a number of "asset mix" questionnaires on the Internet that purport to give guidance on the types of investments you should be considering. Use these tools as a guide, but be aware of their limitations. Focus on those Web sites that provide useful educational information about the concept of asset allocation.

- The Internet can assist you in preparing your investment objective statement and determining an appropriate asset mix whether or not you use a financial planner or advisor.

When it comes right down to it, various investments have different characteristics—some are riskier than others but have a good potential to grow in value, while others have very little risk and a solid stream of income but no potential for growth in its overall value. However, every investment has a certain combination of risk, income, and growth characteristics (a topic we discuss in appendix B, "Basic Investment Concepts").

To decide how you should invest, you should determine the type of investor you are. Are you risk adverse? Are you looking for long-term growth in the value of your investments—and are you willing to subject yourself to a little more risk to help accomplish that? Or do you need a solid stream of income from your investments right now and therefore can accept little risk?

All of these things need to be considered when trying to answer the next two questions:

- What are my investment objectives; what is the goal I am trying to reach?

- What specific investments will I need in my investment portfolio to help meet my investment objectives?

When determining your investment objectives you need to understand two basic concepts: diversification and asset mix.

- Diversification means that you should put your money into a range of different types of investments. It is extremely important that you diversify your portfolio.

- Developing your own asset mix means determining what assets (investments) to hold and how much of each type. To do this you need to educate yourself on the risk, income, and growth characteristics of different types of investments.

Combining these concepts is how you determine what to invest in. There is one caution that we have for you, however—everyone has a theory!

Everyone Has a Theory

As you plunge further and further into the world of investing, you will quickly realize that everyone has a theory about the best way to decide what you should invest in. Here are three examples:

- Some financial experts live and die by the statistical formulas they use to rank various investments. In the mutual fund industry, many experts go to great lengths to assign a numerical ranking to each and every mutual fund, based on a series of elaborate calculations involving the various characteristics of the fund. They believe that this scientific approach to investing helps investors make the best decisions.

- Others research the past performance of investments and use numerical ranking methods to figure out the best investments. With mutual funds, this is done through an exhaustive examination of mutual fund tables in order to highlight the best performers. With stocks, these analysts chart all kinds of aspects of past performance. Some people who ascribe to this theory believe that the best recent performer is likely a good target for investment, while others believe that longer-term performance is a better indicator of potential future performance.

- In the mutual funds industry, some people make their investment decisions based on the track record of the fund managers. In other words, they place their investments with fund managers who have successful track records, and they avoid fund managers whose track records aren't so stellar.

> ...investment advisers have this bit of advice: be prudent. Past returns are no indication of future performance. And everyone should be prepared for lower returns, or even a drop after three years of high returns on equities.
>
> SUSAN NOAKES, "MUTUAL STAMPEDE—DOUBLE-DIGIT RETURNS ON EQUITY FUNDS LOOK ENTICING, BUT EXPERTS ADVISE PRUDENCE," *FINANCIAL POST*, FEBRUARY 1, 1997

There is probably a degree of merit to each of these theories. But regardless of what types of investments you're considering, there's no one best solution and no quick route to success.

We think this is an important point to raise, because as you travel through the Internet you will encounter an often overwhelming number of investment theories. You'll read all kinds of information and discover a number of people who indicate that they have the "definitive" or "best" answer when it comes to learning how to invest.

We think you should keep in mind this basic fact—a theory is just a theory, and when it comes to investing, everyone has a theory. No theory is foolproof.

The Need for Diversification!

Even though there are all kinds of theories about how to decide what to invest in, most financial experts agree on one simple, basic principle: when investing, whether for your retirement or otherwise, you should spread your investment money across a variety of different types of investment.

This is another way of saying that you shouldn't place all of your eggs in one basket.

This strategy allows you to have a range of investments with different risk, growth, and income characteristics in your overall investment plan.

At the same time, they will also advise you not to invest in too many things—don't carry too many eggs in your basket! Most professionals would say that a well-diversified portfolio consists of anywhere from five to ten different types of investments, but not more; otherwise, you are making things far too complex.

This is called diversification—a basic but significant investment strategy.

Examples of Diversification

Now, you might say, "Why would you want to do that?" Let's explain the reasons for diversification using three examples.

First, let's say that you are the type of investor who is willing to live with quite a bit of risk in the types of investments that you are going to make because you really want to see some growth in the value of your overall investment. You decide to place all of your investment money in the stock market—whether directly or by way of mutual funds that invest in stocks. If the stock market suffers a major upheaval, you will probably lose a good chunk of money. On the other hand, if you had invested at least some of your investment money in cash-based securities, as well as some in stock-based investments, you would be safer, since the cash-based investments won't fall in price when the stock market falls.

Second, let's say that you are the type of investor who does not feel comfortable with any sort of risk and therefore have placed all of your investment money in cash-based securities. You'll have a very secure investment portfolio, but you will not see much of an increase in the value of your investment over time, since cash-based securities generally have no growth element attached to them. If you had put at least some of your investment money into stock-based investments, you could share in some of the growth that can come from an increase in the value of such investments.

Third, let's say that income is your most important investment objective. You place all of your money in blue chip stocks and earn a regular stream of income in the form of dividends. But over time you don't share in any of the spectacular growth that is occurring with the share values of small companies—so while you have steady income, the overall value of your investments isn't increasing. Instead, if you place a small percentage—say, 10% or 20%—of your overall investment in the stock of such small companies, you'll still get the regular income from the balance of your investments that are held in blue chip stocks, while obtaining some investment growth from those smaller stocks.

Diversification means that you want to have a mix of assets in your investment portfolio. You should invest in a mix of investments, each of which is different in terms of its income, risk, and growth profile.

Educate Yourself

We think that your first step to figuring out your asset mix should be to use the Internet to do some *basic* research on the risk, growth, and income characteristics of different investments.

You really need to understand clearly that different types of investments will serve different purposes for

> **Carlson On-line (www.carlsononline.com)** is probably one of the most comprehensive sites when it comes to Canadian investment information. It features over 50,000 links organized by company. All Canadian public companies on the Toronto Stock Exchange, the Montreal Stock Exchange, the Alberta Stock Exchange, the Vancouver Stock Exchange, and the Canadian Dealer Network are included. Simply enter a stock symbol or part of the company name, and the search engine will provide a single page of links appropriate for that company. Links include:
> - press releases from a blended feed from Canadian NewsWire, Canadian Corporate News, and the Information Service Dissemination Network
> - corporate Web sites (over 1,600 at last count) and corporate e-mail contacts
> - research reports (if available)
> - links to SEDAR (System for Electronic Document Analysis and Retrieval) for annual reports, financial statements, and prospectuses
> - links for delayed quotes and charts
> - links to the exchange Web sites where appropriate
> - links to discussion groups maintained by Silicon Investor where appropriate
> - links to Strategis (Industry Canada) for industry overviews

you—and with the need for diversification, you need to have several different types of investments.

What should you do? We think you should examine various mutual fund descriptions online to see how they are described in terms of risk, growth, and income. Spend some time reviewing online information about cash-based investments in order to understand their characteristics. Read about and understand how stocks and bonds fluctuate in value—which you can often do simply by reading many financial reports online. You do not need to review every investment or mutual fund that exists, only enough to give you a good understanding of the characteristics of each type of investment.

When it comes to mutual funds, remember that you want to learn about the following:

CHAPTER 3: Determining What to Invest In

- First, use the Internet to learn more about the basic categories of mutual funds—equity, bond/income, money market, mortgage, dividend, resource, specialty, and balanced funds. Reexamine the types of investments held in such funds, where the return comes from, and the risk profile associated with each investment. In light of your own circumstances, what seems most appropriate for you? Which ones interest you, and which ones make you too nervous? Jot down a preliminary list of the various fund categories that are most appropriate for you, keeping in mind you are trying to figure out where particular types of funds fit in with your investment objectives.

- Second, take some time to learn more about the funds available within these particular fund categories by using the Internet. Visit the Web sites for particular mutual funds as we describe later in this book, and seek out several examples of each fund category. For example, examine the descriptions and objectives for a few equity funds, and look at the descriptions for a few mortgage funds, and the same for every other fund category. What are the characteristics of the various categories and types in terms of risk, income, and growth? Which particular types within a category meet your objectives?

- Third, take some time to learn how particular funds fluctuate in light of the investments held in the fund. When reading the online descriptions, take a look at the investments that a particular company has placed its money in. You will find that most Web sites offer details about the major investments held in a fund. For example, if you look at an equity fund, you will see that you can obtain a list of the largest holdings in the fund. Think about how the value of the fund could change in the future in light of this information.

- Fourth, work with some of the online analysis tools such as GLOBEfund that we describe in chapter 6. These tools will help you understand how a particular type of fund fluctuates in value compared to other types of funds or in comparison to other factors such as the performance of the stock market.

- Fifth, use these same tools to help you identify funds that have particularly good or particularly poor histories over the long term, to understand more about their growth potential. You will find that services like GLOBEfund and PALTrak, which we discuss in chapters 6 and 9, permit you to analyze the performance of funds. They also allow you to highlight particularly good performers, which is useful when you actually begin to decide which funds to invest in.

By doing this type of background research before it is time to figure out a specific asset mix for you, you'll have learned more about what is involved and have a better understanding of what types of investments make sense for you.

Asset Mix

You will continually encounter the concept of diversification as you deal with the investment world. You will hear terms such as "diversification strategy," "investment mix," "asset mix," "asset allocation," and many other similar terms.

All of these terms have to do with the basic investment premise that you should invest your money so that it is in a variety of investments that have different levels of risk, income potential, and growth potential.

> **The asset allocation approach is a long-term strategy that has been proven to be effective to reduce overall risk and increase one's overall rate of return.**
> DEB MACPHERSON, "ASSET ALLOCATION BEST WAY TO START INVESTING," *THE HAMILTON SPECTATOR*, DECEMBER 2, 1996

Your "asset mix," or the different types of investments you will have, is directly determined by your investment objectives.

By determining your investment objectives you can figure out what your asset mix should be. Your asset mix is usually expressed in the form of a percentage of your total investment that you will place in various investment types.

Here's one example of a well-balanced investment objective: you might want an investment portfolio that has a good opportunity for growth in the value of your stocks, yet pays a consistent income and leaves at least some money in very low-risk investments.

To meet these objectives, you might establish an asset mix as follows: you decide to place 25% of your investment money into some blue chip stocks that pay a consistent income in the form of dividends, another 50% into medium-risk, medium growth-potential investments, and the remaining 25% in low-risk, low-growth, cash-based investments. That's a good way of describing your asset mix.

Online Questionnaires

Next, spend a little bit of time with several of the online asset mix questionnaires that you can find on the Internet—while recognizing the clear limitations of these tools.

Throughout the Internet, particularly at the sites of mutual fund companies, you will come across many online questionnaires that appear to simplify your investment decisions. These are called "asset mix" or "asset allocation" questionnaires, since they help you determine the mix of mutual fund assets that you should purchase—and, hence, purport to help you figure out an asset mix that is just right for you.

Answer the questions, and you will receive a suggested asset mix. Thus, you can use these tools as a useful step toward understanding your investment objectives and asset mix.

Try Out a Few Mutual Fund Asset Mix Tools

First, try out some of the mutual fund asset questionnaires to be found online.

Take a look at how it works. You answer some simple questions about your attitude toward mutual funds, investing, risk, and other factors.

1999 MUTUAL FUNDS AND RRSPs ONLINE

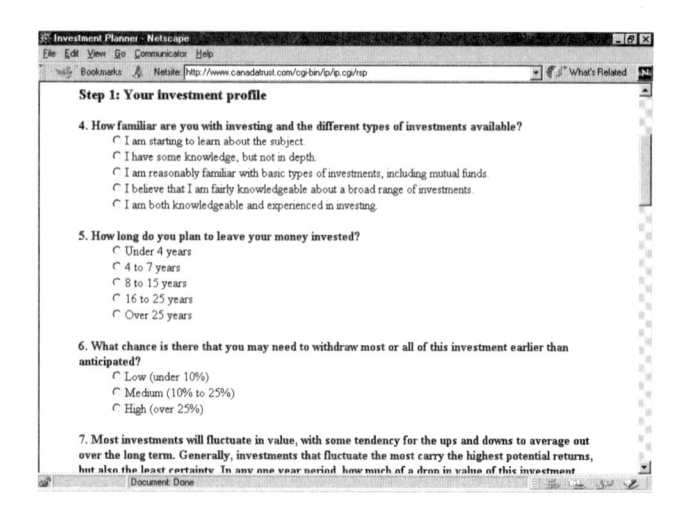

> **Step 1: Your investment profile**
>
> **4. How familiar are you with investing and the different types of investments available?**
> ○ I am starting to learn about the subject.
> ○ I have some knowledge, but not in depth.
> ○ I am reasonably familiar with basic types of investments, including mutual funds.
> ○ I believe that I am fairly knowledgeable about a broad range of investments.
> ○ I am both knowledgeable and experienced in investing.
>
> **5. How long do you plan to leave your money invested?**
> ○ Under 4 years
> ○ 4 to 7 years
> ○ 8 to 15 years
> ○ 16 to 25 years
> ○ Over 25 years
>
> **6. What chance is there that you may need to withdraw most or all of this investment earlier than anticipated?**
> ○ Low (under 10%)
> ○ Medium (10% to 25%)
> ○ High (over 25%)
>
> 7. Most investments will fluctuate in value, with some tendency for the ups and downs to average out over the long term. Generally, investments that fluctuate the most carry the highest potential returns, but also the least certainty. In any one year period, how much of a drop in value of this investment

Then, a few seconds later, the site recommends a mix of diversified investments that is "appropriate" for you based on the information you supplied.

Tools such as these are found on many investment Web sites in Canada—you won't have to look far to find a number of them.

But don't make a mistake—you have to be very cautious of such tools.

Take this Canada Trust site as an example. The planner's opening screen says that "in a few seconds, you'll see our recommendations for the right combination of Canada Trust investments designed to meet your goals." You should be suspicious as soon as you see a statement like that—especially once you realize that the suggested asset mix consists mostly of specific mutual funds from Canada Trust.

CHAPTER 3 : Determining What to Invest In

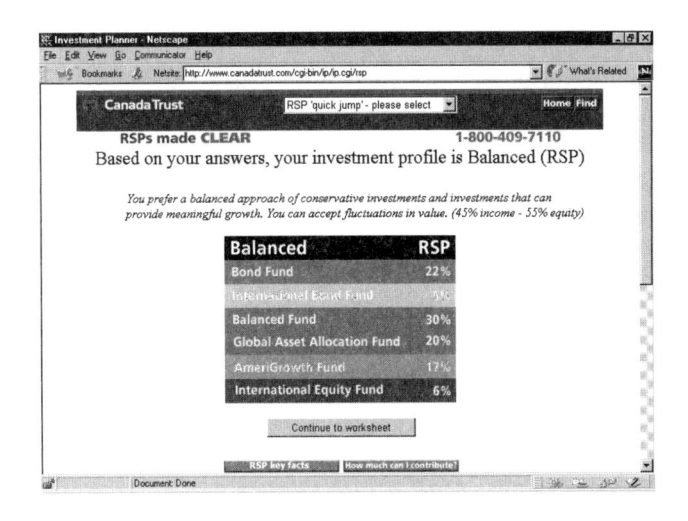

[Screenshot of Canada Trust Investment Planner web page showing:]

RSPs made CLEAR — 1-800-409-7110

Based on your answers, your investment profile is Balanced (RSP)

You prefer a balanced approach of conservative investments and investments that can provide meaningful growth. You can accept fluctuations in value. (45% income - 55% equity)

Balanced	RSP
Bond Fund	22%
International Equity Fund	5%
Balanced Fund	30%
Global Asset Allocation Fund	20%
AmeriGrowth Fund	17%
International Equity Fund	6%

This appears to be a listing of mutual fund types that you should invest in, but examine it carefully. It is suggesting specific Canada Trust mutual funds, for example, AmeriGrowth Fund.

The thing about these investment questionnaires is this—while the solutions they present certainly seem to make life simple, they are often too biased to suggest anything other than a rough form of guidance.

After all, it would be wonderful if our complex investment decisions could be simplified by answering a few questions. Unfortunately, investment decisions aren't that easy. We'll discuss this issue in greater depth below.

Try Out a Few General Asset Mix Tools

We find that the mutual fund questionnaires, such as the one seen above, are very biased. Having said that, there are some financial Web sites that provide asset mix information in a manner that is far more even-handed.

Rather than telling you which specific funds or investments to buy, they offer guidance on the types of mutual fund investments you should be considering.

For example, definitely spend some time on the Financial Pipeline Web site. It promotes itself as an independent source of investment information, where "all articles are screened and edited for accuracy and impartiality." Sponsored by such companies as C.T. Private Investment Counsel and the Canadian Bond Rating Service, the site features an extensive selection of useful

1999 MUTUAL FUNDS AND RRSPs ONLINE

background information on a wide variety of mutual fund topics, including a number of articles about asset mix decisions.

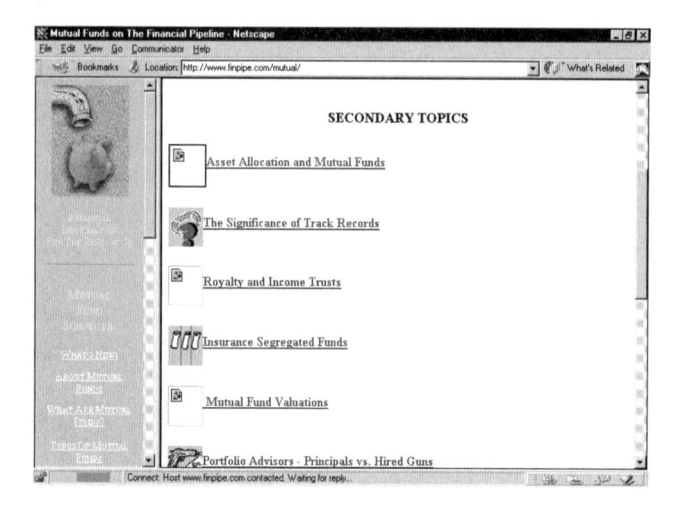

At the Canada Life Web site, you can fill out an "Investor Type Profiler" questionnaire that will help you assess what type of investor you are and what type of portfolio would best suit your investing style.

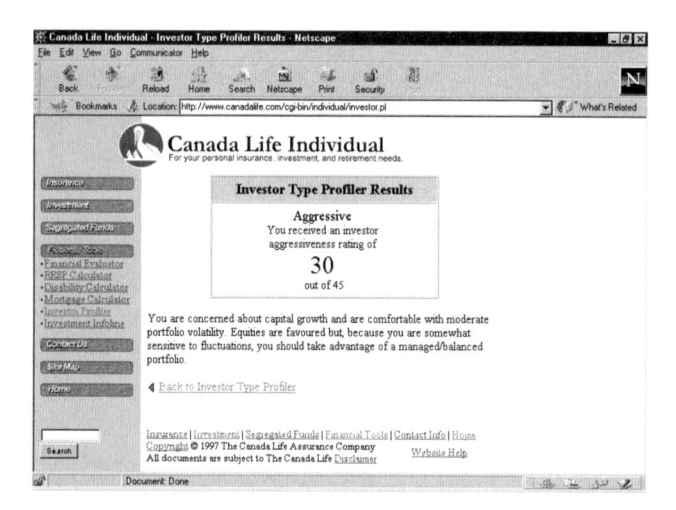

Citizens Bank of Canada has a similar tool entitled "RRSP Questionnaire." Although it refers to RRSP investments, the questions and results can be used for non-RRSP investments as well.

CHAPTER 3 : Determining What to Invest In

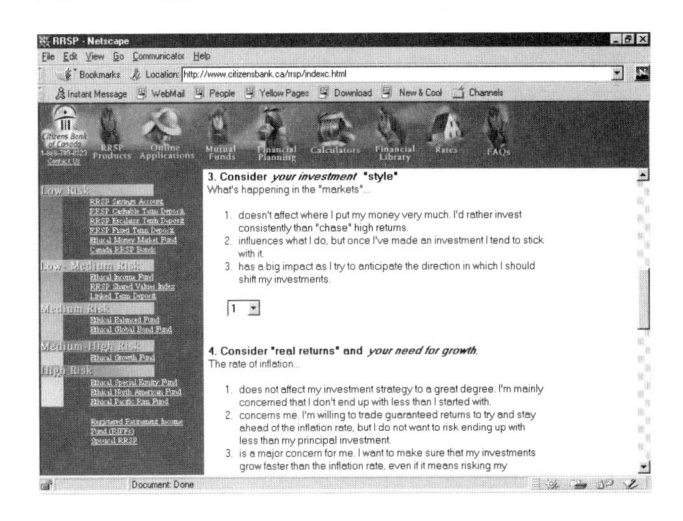

For some good background information on the issues that might affect your asset allocation, visit ilmoney and have look at the Knowledge Base section. There you will find good articles such as "Setting Your Investment Goals" and "Determining Your Risk Profile."

Similarly, at Quicken.ca you'll find useful information in the Investing for Beginners section. In particular, take a look at the article "Why you invest tells you how to invest."

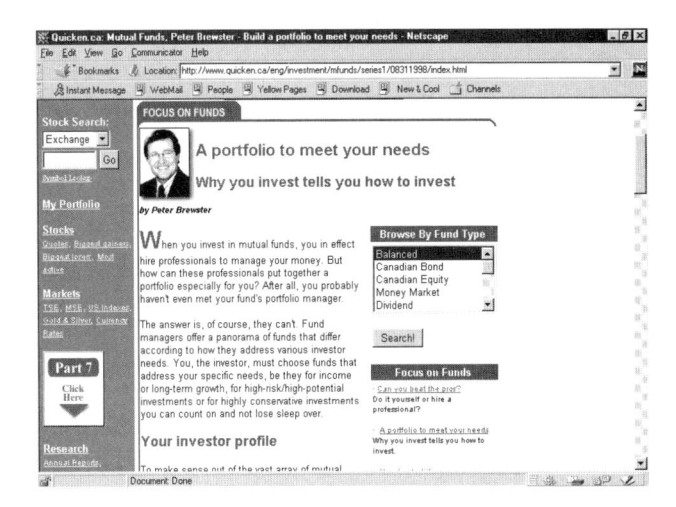

Also visit the investment section of *The Vancouver Sun*'s Web site. You'll find it under the Business category. They have an excellent investment area that includes information on how to decide what to invest in.

53

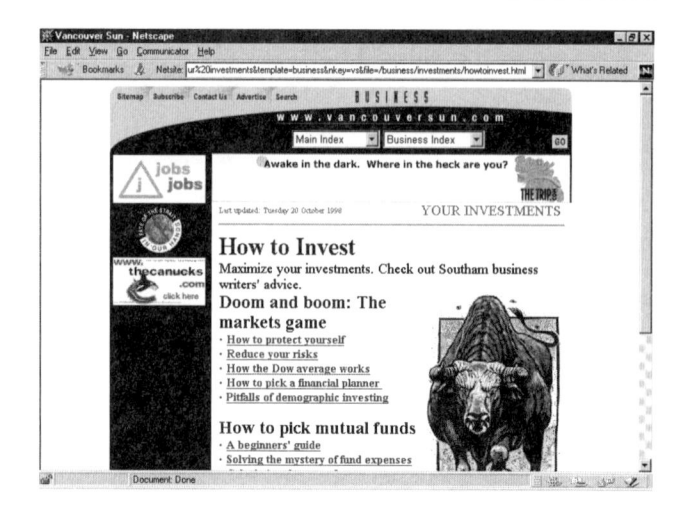

Recognize the Limitations of These Tools

What's the bottom line? We suggest that you experiment with the asset mix questionnaires you find on the Internet, but use them with caution. We also suggest that you use a number of them to see how their answers differ.

While mutual fund asset mix questionnaires can provide general guidance on the types of funds you should consider—such as equity, bond, or mortgage funds—they should not and cannot serve as a definitive answer to your investment needs.

We think playing around with these tools can be useful—but we also think that you shouldn't fall into the trap of thinking that they provide a definitive answer to what is essentially a very complicated question. While asset mix questionnaires are a tremendously powerful marketing tool, they really can't give you a good, accurate indication of where you should be investing your money. First of all, they often simplify what are really complex financial decisions. In addition, they are often biased toward the financial institution administering the questionnaire.

We find that asset mix questionnaires fall prey to the "we'll-suggest-what-we-sell" syndrome. For example, after you answer the questions, the final recommendation is usually that you buy the investments offered by the financial institution that prepared the questionnaire. But this should come as no great surprise because the firm obviously isn't going to refer you to any of its competitors. Naturally, they are going to recommend their own funds.

CHAPTER 3 : Determining What to Invest In

Your Investment Objectives

Now that you've spent time learning more about the characteristics of different investments and have considered some of the online asset mix tools that are available to get some guidance on your own investment needs, it's time to bite the bullet and write down your investment objectives. Establishing your investment objectives in the form of a single paragraph is perhaps the most difficult thing for you to do—but is an absolute necessity.

> **Want to learn about investing with little risk? Many online brokerages allow you to join a "game" online in which you buy and sell various investments over a period of time. In particular, take a look at E*Trade Canada (www.canada.etrade.com) and Quicken.ca (www.quicken.ca).**

Many financial planners and investment advisors can help you figure out your investment objectives and assist you in coming up with an asset mix based on these objectives.

Often, their advice can be well worth the fee that they will charge you—they have the expertise, background, and historical track record to help you figure out what you want to accomplish with your investments, and can translate that into an easily understood investment objective. From that, they can assist you in establishing a good, diversified mix of different types of assets that will help you achieve those objectives.

Still many people decide to figure out their investment objectives and therefore their asset mix on their own.

There is no simpler way to go through this than to write out your objectives. Carefully balance what you think you need in terms of growth in your investment portfolio, your attitudes toward risk, and what you might need in terms of income.

Here is an example of what we mean:

> I am investing for my retirement for the long term. I'll therefore place the majority of my investments in assets that have a good long-term potential for growth.

I'm willing to take some risk with these long-term investments, but not a great deal. I'll also ensure that I have a ready source of cash available, so I'll place some of my money in cash-based investments so that I can access it if needed. Since I'm investing for my retirement, I don't really need to focus on investments that provide a regular stream of income in the short term.

You must prepare the same type of statement—and you can only do this by sitting back and thinking about what you really want to accomplish. There isn't much the Internet can do here to help you—you can only do this through some long, careful thinking on your part.

Figuring Out Your Asset Mix

Finally, you will need to translate this investment objective statement into a definitive asset mix.

Keep in mind that the percentages we use below are examples—what is right for you depends on your own investment objectives.

First, figure out what percentage of your overall investment holdings should be in cash-based holdings, recognizing that you always want to have some percentage of your investments in this low-risk category. This might include GICs, CSBs, or term deposits; mutual funds that invest in these types of cash-based investments; or a combination of both. You might decide, for example, to ensure that 20%–25% of your total investment portfolio includes cash-based investments.

Second, diversification means that you should have a mix of different types of investments for the remaining 75%–80%. So you have to figure out, in terms of percentages, how the rest of your investment portfolio should be allocated among different types of investments. What percentage should go into investments that have a good opportunity for growth but are high risk? Medium risk and medium growth? Low risk and low growth?

You might decide to place 20%–25% of your money in high-risk investments, another 30%–35% in medium-risk investments, and the remaining 20%–25% in investments that provide a consistent income with low risk.

Your asset mix percentages would then look something like this:

- 20%–25% cash-based investments
- 20%–25% high risk
- 30%–35% medium risk
- 20%–25% income investments

Now you have to figure out what investments to place in each of these categories.

There is no magic answer to figuring out your investment asset mix in terms of percentages as expressed above. Nor is there an easy way to figure out what investments are appropriate in each of these categories. What it really comes down to is some basic and hard thinking about what your investment objectives are and what asset mix is appropriate to help you meet your objectives.

Always remember this: there is no definitive, absolutely right, correct answer—it is all a matter of judgment.

The Role of the Internet with Your Investments

Can the Internet help you to determine what investments are appropriate for you so that you meet you investment objectives?

Certainly you can use it to research possible investments and obtain guidance on the types of investments you should consider. But in the final analysis, the Internet is only a tool. Your judgment and analysis of your investment objectives and of particular investments are key to discerning what best suits you, in light of the risk, growth, and income specifics that you are willing to accept.

In the next several chapters we will show you how you can use the Internet as a tool to learn more about cash-based investments, mutual funds, and other investments. But first we'll examine some of the tools you can use to assess your current retirement situation.

Web Sites Mentioned in This Chapter

Canada Life	www.canadalife.com
Canada Trust	www.canadatrust.com
Citizens Bank of Canada	www.citizensbank.ca
Financial Pipeline	www.finpipe.com
GLOBEfund	www.globefund.com
ilmoney	www.imoney.com
PALTrak	www.pal.com
Quicken.ca	www.quicken.ca
The Vancouver Sun	www.vancouversun.com

CHAPTER 4

Using Financial Calculators

If something is so complicated that you can't explain it in 10 seconds, then it's probably not worth knowing anyway. CALVIN AND HOBBES

HIGHLIGHTS

- Many Web sites feature financial calculators that will help you manage your RRSPs and plan for your retirement.

- These financial calculators can be used to answer five fundamental questions:

    How much money will I need to retire comfortably?

    How much money will I need to save each year to meet my retirement goals?

    What tax savings will my RRSP contribution generate?

    Should I borrow to contribute to my RRSP?

    Should I contribute to my RRSP or pay down my mortgage?

- Exercise caution when using financial calculators. They work under a certain set of assumptions that may or may not be valid for your particular financial situation.

When it comes to retirement planning on the Internet, we find the many retirement and RRSP "calculators" now available to be most useful.

These tools put into perspective, often dramatically, some of the important concepts related to saving for your retirement. Many of these calculators will serve as a wake-up call, helping you to quickly determine that retirement planning is not something that you should put off.

Play around with these calculators and you will quickly discover how much money you should be putting away today to retire comfortably in the future or how much tax you will save by contributing to an RRSP this year. Some online calculators will also let you assess aspects of your expected financial position upon retirement.

Five Important Financial Questions

In any material that you read about retirement planning there is one piece of advice that is always repeated: do not delay in saving for your retirement. Showing you why you shouldn't delay is an area where the Internet can really be a great help.

Many financial institutions and other organizations provide financial calculators on their Web sites. These calculators help you understand how much you need to save to retire, what level of income you can expect upon retirement, and how much money you will save with a certain RRSP contribution.

Using such calculators will, more than anything else, hammer home the importance of starting to save for your retirement as soon as possible.

How Much Money Will I Need to Retire Comfortably?

The First Canadian Mutual Funds Web site, for example, provides a "retirement planner" (found under the "Investment tools" section) that helps you prepare a cash flow projection. This will help you figure out how much money you will have coming in and going out during your retirement. It is a good starting point for determining how much income you will need to retire comfortably.

CHAPTER 4: Using Financial Calculators

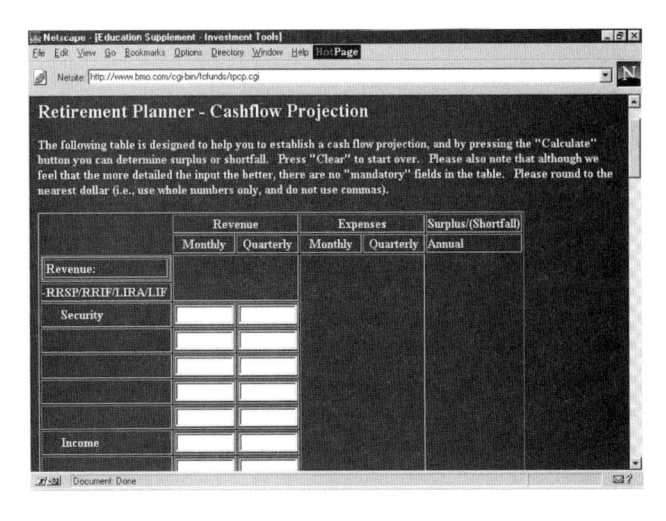

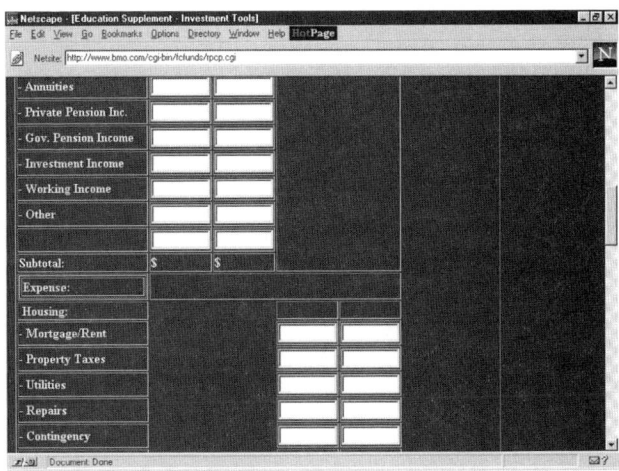

LOOKING FOR OTHER FINANCIAL CALCULATORS?

Strangely enough, you should check out the site for The Institute of Biological Engineering (www.ibe.web.org). Under the category IBE Web Resources, and then IBE Tools, you'll find an entry for Online calculators. From there, you can discover all kinds of tools, including many financial calculators, some of which are specifically Canadian. In addition, do a search for the phrase "RRSP calculators" on a search engine such as AltaVista, and you'll be rewarded with an extensive list.

While not an online calculator, the AGF Group of Funds has a handy worksheet on its Web site that you can use to figure out how much income you will need when you retire. You'll need a calculator or spreadsheet to use it.

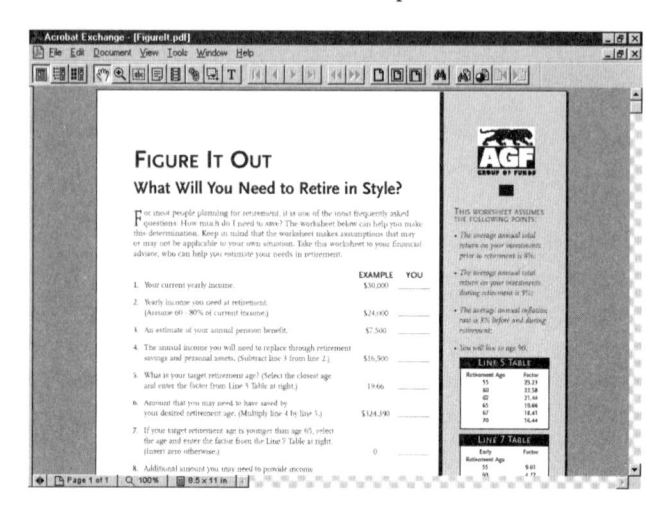

Obviously, such tools are not definitive, but they will get you thinking about the types of expenses that you will be faced with upon retirement and the level of income you will require to meet those expenses.

Knowing what level of income you need is critical to determining the answer to the next question—how much do you need to save this year and each and every other year that follows?

How Much Money Will I Need to Save Each Year to Meet My Retirement Goals?

Not only will the Web help you understand how much you need to save now to retire comfortably in the future, it will help you appreciate the time value of money.

For example, Altamira Investment Services has an RRSP calculator on its Web site that you can use to determine how much you will have to save each year in order to retire with a certain income in the future. Using such a tool will help you to realize what you need to be doing today in order to adequately plan for your retirement.

To use the calculator, you need to supply some figures, such as the value of your current RRSP holdings, your desired retirement income, the rate of return you expect to earn annually on your RRSP investments, and other

CHAPTER 4 : Using Financial Calculators

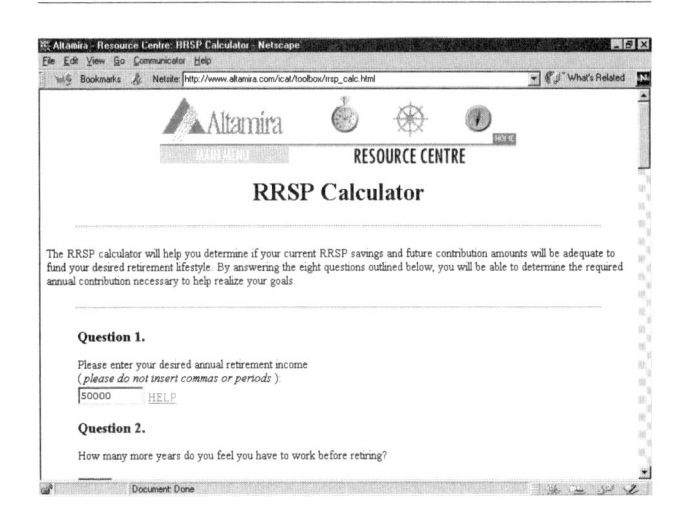

information. If you need assistance filling out the form, you can access an online help screen.

Once you've filled in all the required information, you are provided with a simple and straightforward report that describes how much you will have to contribute to your RRSP each year in order to meet your goals.

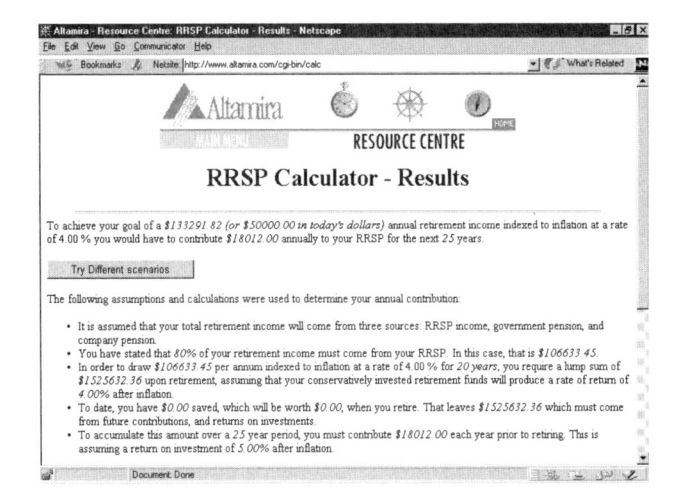

Dynamic Mutual Funds provides a similar calculator on its Web site (see following page). It helps you understand what you need to contribute to an RRSP and how much you need to invest in non-RRSP savings, in order to retire with a certain level of income in the future.

One of the most important fundamentals of saving for your retirement is recognizing the importance of starting

1999 MUTUAL FUNDS AND RRSPs ONLINE

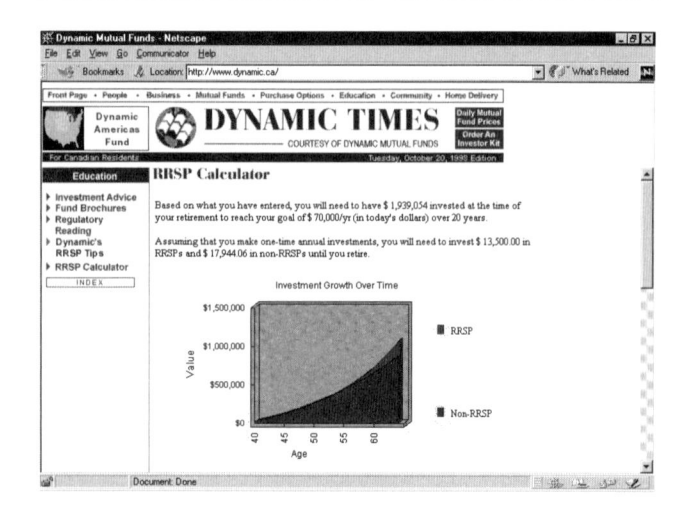

to save earlier rather than later. This concept is best illustrated by using an Internet calculator that helps you to understand the importance of time when contributing to an RRSP.

The Mutual Group provides just such a calculator. Provide the calculator with information on your current salary, age, and amount you'd like to contribute monthly to an RRSP, and it will calculate the retirement income that will be available to you at the age of sixty-five. It tells you how your situation would differ should you decide to wait five or ten years before starting to invest in your RRSP.

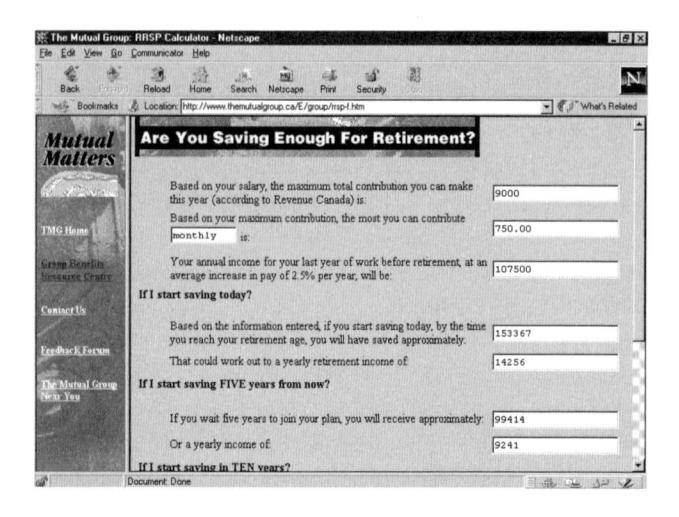

What Tax Savings Will My RRSP Contribution Generate?

Another important issue is knowing how much tax you will save by making a contribution to your RRSP.

Ernst & Young Canada has a calculator on its Web site that tells you how much of a tax saving you can expect from your RRSP contribution. Simply provide the form with your taxable income and RRSP contribution, and the site will calculate the tax savings you can expect to receive in each Canadian province and territory.

> You can find a wealth of financial calculators at the two Canadian financial supersites, Quicken.ca (www.quicken.ca) and iImoney (www.imoney.com).

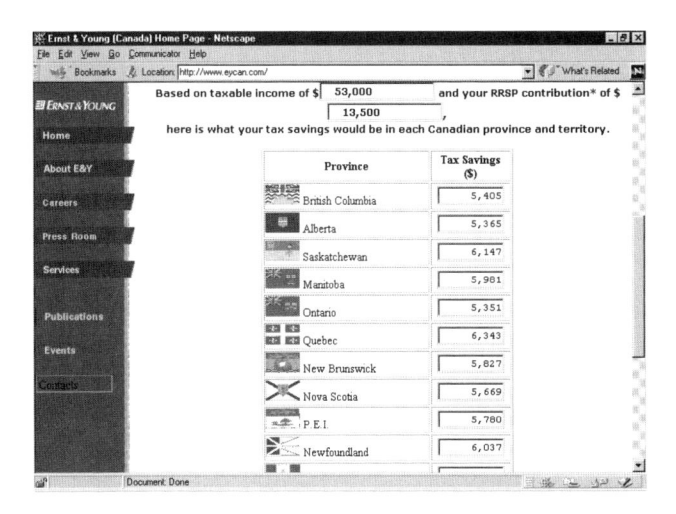

Based on taxable income of $53,000 and your RRSP contribution* of $13,500, here is what your tax savings would be in each Canadian province and territory.

Province	Tax Savings ($)
British Columbia	5,405
Alberta	5,365
Saskatchewan	6,147
Manitoba	5,981
Ontario	5,351
Quebec	6,343
New Brunswick	5,827
Nova Scotia	5,669
P.E.I.	5,780
Newfoundland	6,037

Should I Borrow to Contribute to My RRSP?

It sometimes makes sense to borrow money to invest in an RRSP. The tax implications of doing so are generally in your favour.

The Scotiabank Web site (see following page) includes a calculator that you can use to see the benefits of taking out a loan to contribute to your RRSP.

1999 MUTUAL FUNDS AND RRSPs ONLINE

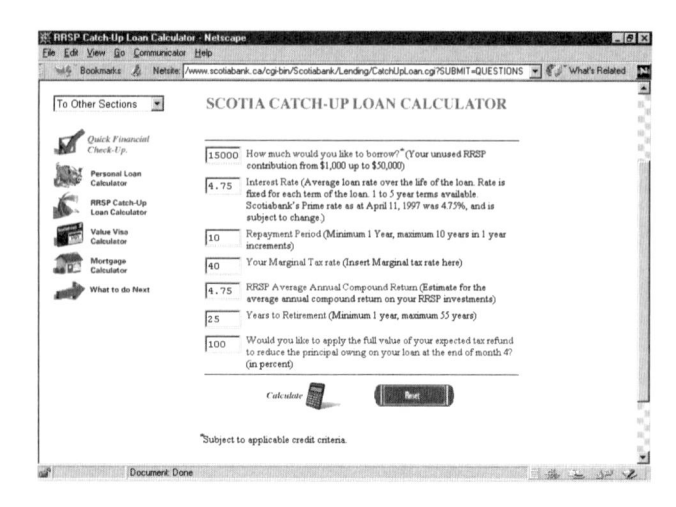

Should I Contribute to My RRSP or Pay Down My Mortgage?

A dilemma that many Canadians face is whether to invest any extra money they might have in an RRSP, or whether it should be used to pay down their mortgage.

RetireWeb includes a calculator that can help you make this important decision. First, provide the calculator with information about the extra money you have, your tax rate, your mortgage rate, and other factors.

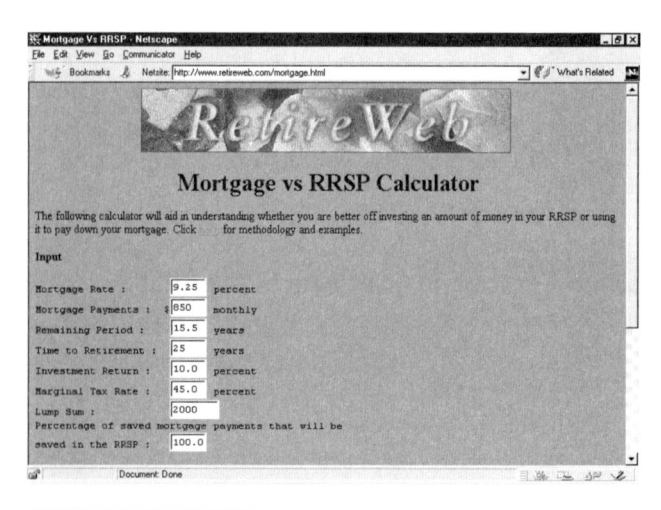

> **Another useful source for Canadian financial information is the Sympatico site (www.sympatico.ca). Take a look at the personal finance section: there are more than fifteen very useful financial calculators.**

Based on the information you supply, the calculator presents its recommendation. An example is seen on the screen below. If you need more information about the recommendation, read the information screen that the Web site provides.

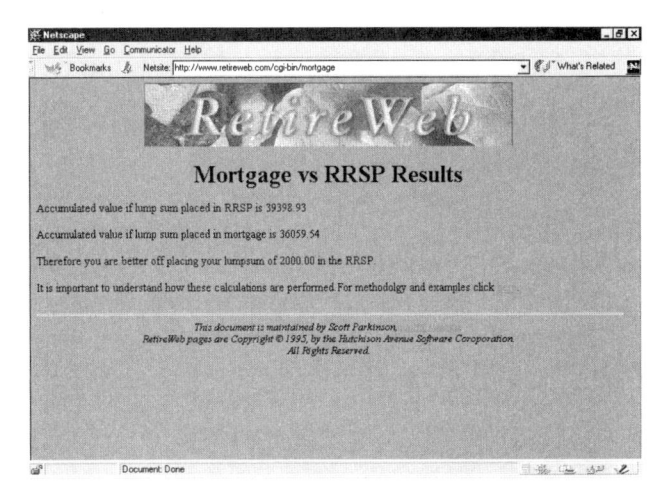

The Emergence of Sophisticated Planning Tools

Finally, as you use many of these calculators, you will find some that are more sophisticated than others. Many calculators are starting to provide a lot of flexibility in the way that you can analyze your retirement options.

Scotiabank's Web site, for instance, features an interactive tool called the Scotiabank Reality Check. It can be used to determine whether you will be able to meet your retirement goals based on your current level of RRSP savings.

1999 MUTUAL FUNDS AND RRSPs ONLINE

As an example, the screen below shows a report for a hypothetical Internet user. The next screen indicates the shortfall that will result from an inadequate investment in an RRSP, based on the person's current income and RRSP investment levels.

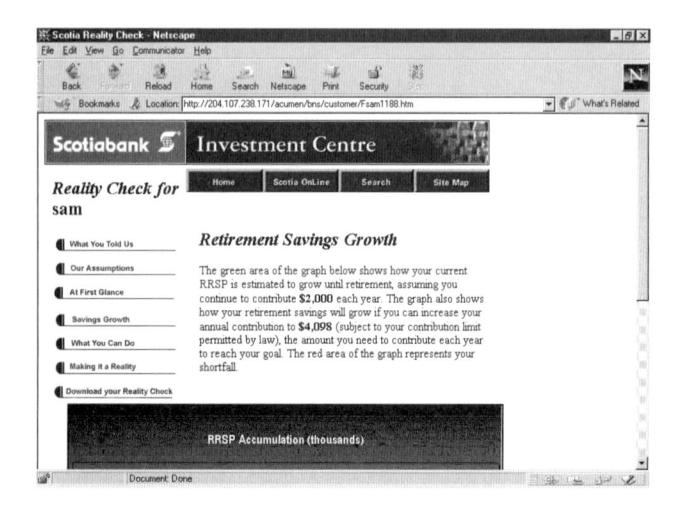

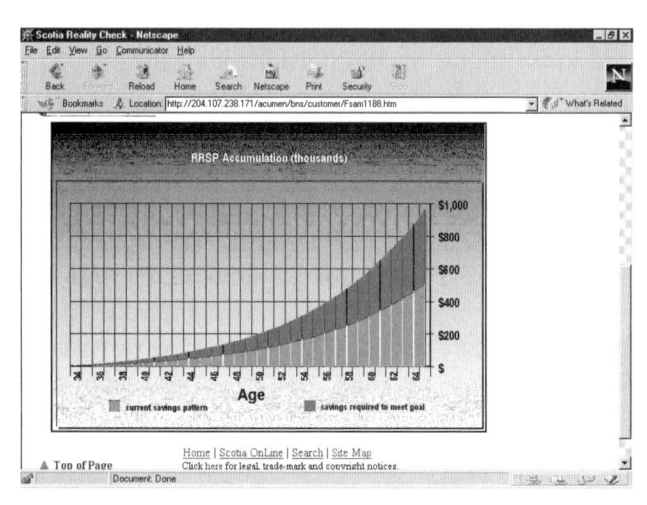

Spend a bit of time in this particular Web site, and you can "play" with many different retirement scenarios—and truly appreciate the necessity for action on your part.

Similarly, Canada Trust's Web site lets you examine multiple scenarios that might affect your retirement plans, helping you to better understand the impact of varying levels of retirement savings.

CHAPTER 4 : Using Financial Calculators

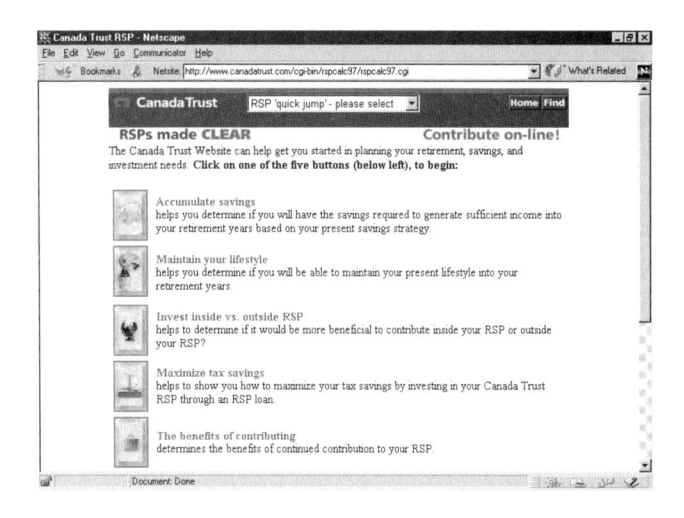

The key point is this: using the Internet to help you understand RRSP and retirement issues can be extremely beneficial, for it can help to bring some realism to the questions that you are struggling with.

Two Final Hints

As you use the calculators described in this chapter, we suggest that you take the time to double-check their math. If you find calculators on different Web sites that perform the same function, it wouldn't hurt to check your numbers in each of them to see if they match. After all, these are computers that we are dealing with, and computer calculations aren't necessarily always 100% reliable.

In addition, most financial calculators operate under a certain set of assumptions. These assumptions may or may not be applicable to your particular financial situation.

The bottom line is to always question the information you obtain from the Internet, even if it is a tool such as those described in this chapter. Financial calculators aren't a substitute for sound financial advice. Check with a financial advisor or financial professional before acting on any of the results provided by a financial calculator.

Web Sites Mentioned in This Chapter

AGF Group of Funds	www.agf.ca
Altamira Investment Services	www.altamira.com
Canada Trust	www.canadatrust.com
Dynamic Mutual Funds	www.dynamic.ca
Ernst & Young Canada	www.eycan.com
First Canadian Mutual Funds	www.bmo.com/fcfunds
RetireWeb	www.retireweb.com
Scotiabank	www.scotiabank.ca
The Mutual Group	www.themutualgroup.com

CHAPTER 5

Cash and Cash-Equivalent Investments on the Internet

Retirement kills more people than hard work ever did. MALCOLM S. FORBES

HIGHLIGHTS

- Web sites such as CANNEX and CANOE can help you compare interest rates from different banks and trust companies.

- Financial institutions often introduce new variations of existing cash-based investments. You should learn how to do research online to find independent news articles that assess these new cash-based offerings.

- On the Internet, you can research whether your cash-based investments are covered by federal deposit insurance or some other form of deposit insurance.

Whether you are looking for information on investments for inside or outside of your RRSP, the Internet is a good place to start. Investments can be put into three categories: cash and cash-equivalents (this includes savings accounts, CSBs, GICs, and term deposits), mutual funds, and stocks and bonds.

We will discuss mutual funds in chapter 6 and stocks and bonds in chapter 7, but first let's look at cash and cash-equivalent investments.

Given the massive number of Canadian financial institutions that have established Web sites, it is no surprise that you can find a lot of information about their cash-based and cash-equivalent offerings online. If you are unfamiliar with the different types of cash-based investments, we suggest you spend a few minutes reviewing appendix D, "Learning About Investments on the Internet."

Using the Internet to Compare Savings Rates

A drawback to the increasing number of Web sites that are available is that you could spend hours comparing the rates of cash-based investments. Fortunately, there are a few excellent sites to check that cover a lot of ground.

First, check out CANNEX, an organization that has supplied interest rate surveys to the financial world for many years. On their site you can get an extensive list of comparative rates for GICs, term deposits, and deposit accounts.

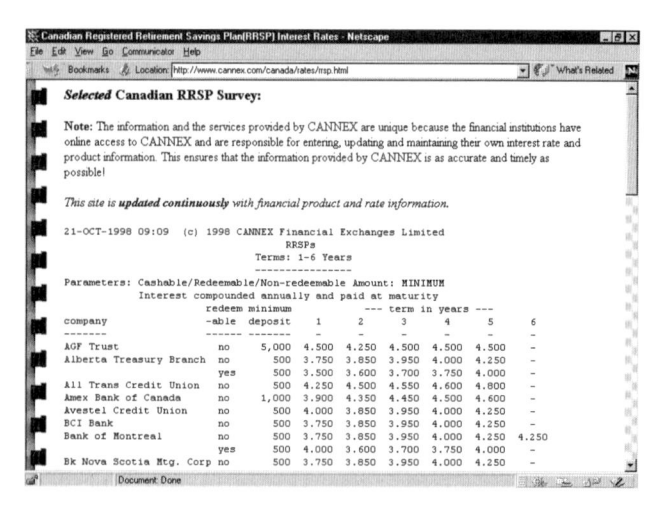

```
Selected Canadian RRSP Survey:

Note: The information and the services provided by CANNEX are unique because the financial institutions have
online access to CANNEX and are responsible for entering, updating and maintaining their own interest rate and
product information. This ensures that the information provided by CANNEX is as accurate and timely as
possible!

This site is updated continuously with financial product and rate information.

21-OCT-1998 09:09   (c) 1998 CANNEX Financial Exchanges Limited
                                     RRSPs
                               Terms: 1-6 Years
                               ----------------
Parameters: Cashable/Redeemable/Non-redeemable Amount: MINIMUM
            Interest compounded annually and paid at maturity
                        redeem minimum            --- term in years ---
company                 -able  deposit   1      2      3      4      5      6
-------                 -----  -------  -----  -----  -----  -----  -----  -----
AGF Trust                no    5,000    4.500  4.250  4.500  4.500  4.500   -
Alberta Treasury Branch  no      500    3.750  3.850  3.950  4.000  4.250   -
                         yes     500    3.500  3.600  3.700  3.750  4.000   -
All Trans Credit Union   no      500    4.250  4.500  4.550  4.600  4.800   -
Amex Bank of Canada      no    1,000    3.900  4.350  4.450  4.500  4.600   -
Avestel Credit Union     no      500    4.000  3.850  3.950  4.000  4.250   -
BCI Bank                 no      500    3.750  3.850  3.950  4.000  4.250   -
Bank of Montreal         no      500    3.750  3.850  3.950  4.000  4.250  4.250
                         yes     500    3.500  3.600  3.700  3.750  4.000   -
Bk Nova Scotia Mtg. Corp no      500    3.750  3.850  3.950  4.000  4.250   -
```

Similarly, the Web sites of ilmoney and Quicken.ca offer pages of detailed comparative interest rates. In Quicken.ca select the Banking category and then choose any of "Savings & Investment Rates" items.

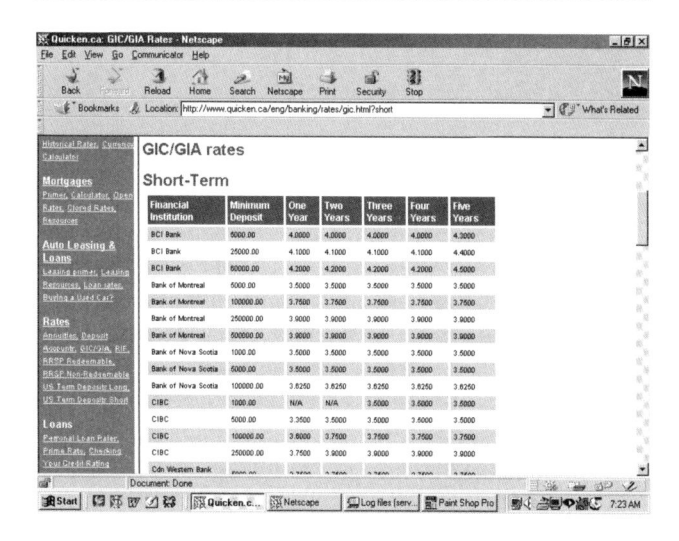

CHAPTER 5: Cash and Cash-Equivalent Investments on the Internet

[Screenshot of Quicken.ca GIC/GIA Rates page showing a table of short-term rates from various financial institutions including BCI Bank, Bank of Montreal, Bank of Nova Scotia, CIBC, and Cdn Western Bank with columns for Minimum Deposit, One Year, Two Years, Three Years, Four Years, and Five Years.]

You can obtain short- and long-term GIC rates, deposit account rates, and even rates for term deposits held in U.S. dollars.

Understanding Innovative Product Offerings

Financial institutions often introduce new variations of basic cash-equivalent accounts in order to make them more attractive to RRSP holders. They often provide details of these new product offerings on their Web sites, such as the example below from the CIBC site.

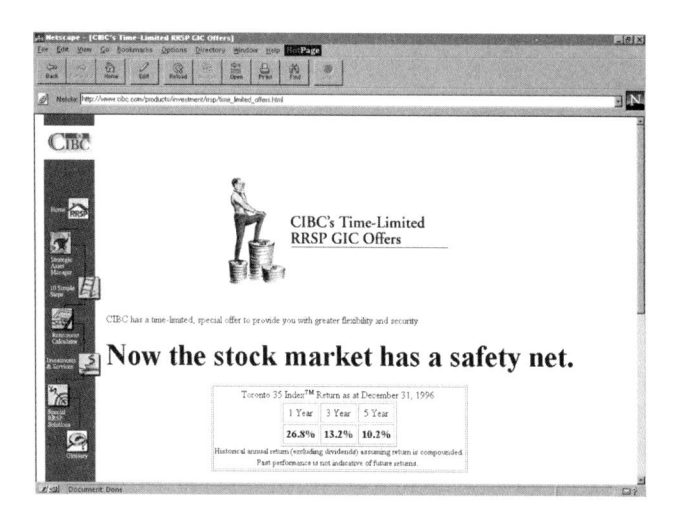

[Screenshot of CIBC's Time-Limited RRSP GIC Offers web page with the headline "Now the stock market has a safety net." and a table showing Toronto 35 Index Return as at December 31, 1996: 1 Year 26.8%, 3 Year 13.2%, 5 Year 10.2%.]

73

> *Computing Canada* estimated that in mid-1998 there were 200,000 online investors in Canada.

You will see many advertisements in newspapers and magazines during RRSP season. You should take the time to use the Internet to learn more about the income, growth, and risk characteristics of the investments being advertised. If the Web site doesn't answer all your questions, you can usually contact the financial organization by e-mail to ask specific questions.

You should also learn to use the Internet to find independent news articles that assess new financial products. Consider the following situation. We received a brochure from the Royal Bank of Canada that promoted a host of new financial products. These new products had names such as:

- Market Rate Increase GIC
- Medical Access GIC
- Canadian Market-Linked GIC
- Global Market-Linked GIC
- Five-in-One GIC
- Building Block GIC
- One-Year Cashable GIC

When you visit the Royal Bank Web site you can certainly learn more about these products. For example, they provide a full page of information about the "Market-Linked GIC," and they describe the benefits associated with this type of investment.

> **Interested in finding out what you might earn on your savings account, GIC, or term deposit? Visit the Hpertechmedia compound interest calculator at hypertechmedia.com/Interest.html—it lets you do lots of quick calculations.**

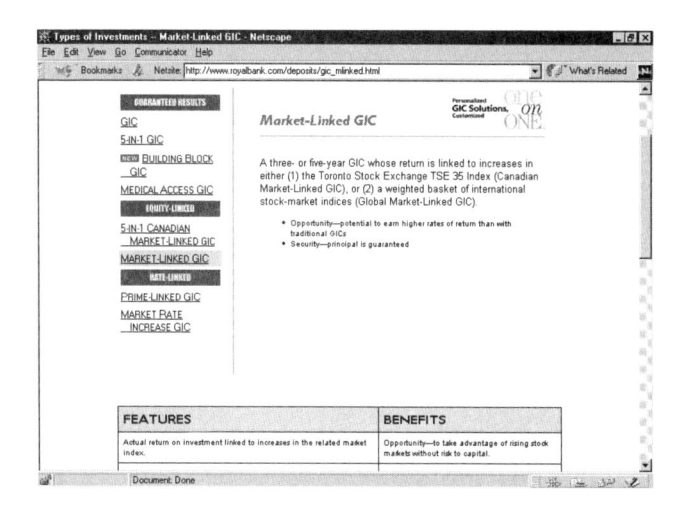

CHAPTER 5 : Cash and Cash-Equivalent Investments on the Internet

On the surface, it sounds like a great, no-lose investment. But what *isn't* clear is the potential risk associated with the product.

To get an independent, unbiased view of these products, you could use the Internet to locate stories in the financial press related to "market-linked GIC" products. How? In our case, we went to the CANOE Web site and did a search for the terms "market-linked" and "GICs."

After a few seconds of searching its database, CANOE returned the search results.

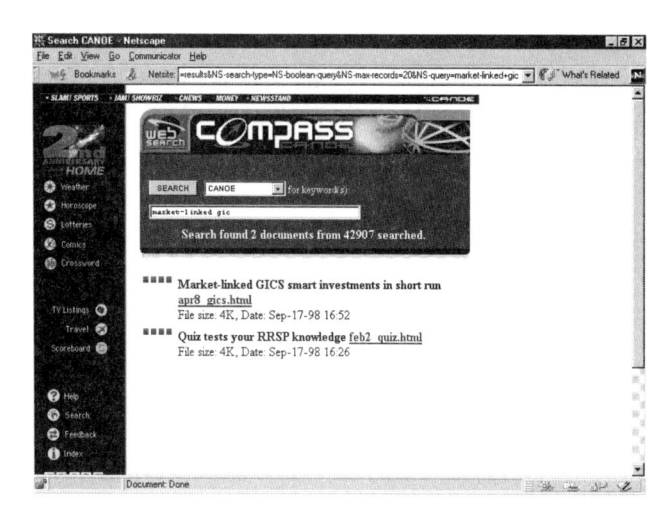

The articles helped us understand that while the basic investment is guaranteed, there is no guarantee of any *income* on the initial investment should the stock market take a significant downturn. That is an important risk to

understand, particularly in these troubled times, but it wasn't clearly identified on the Royal Bank Web site. This example illustrates the importance of balancing the information you obtain online from a financial institution with independent advice from another source such as CANOE.

Many financial institutions aren't as up-front as they should be when it comes to the risk of the financial investments they promote. In some cases, this attitude has carried through to their Web sites.

But any investment carries risk—and the Internet can be a powerful ally to help you learn more about the risk associated with any cash-based financial products you may be considering. The Internet's usefulness as an investment tool extends far beyond the Web sites of financial organizations. It's important to go beyond the online promotional material and research the pros and cons of investments like we did in the example above. Only then will you be able to make a fully informed decision.

The lesson to be learned? Whatever you do, don't plunge into an investment without fully understanding what you are getting into. Learn to use the Internet to uncover the information that the Web site of a financial institution doesn't tell you.

Learning About the Security of Your Investment

It is important to find out whether the financial institution you are dealing with is covered by some type of deposit insurance. This isn't necessarily an easy question to answer online. Many financial institutions don't provide this information on their Web sites.

But some do. For example, here is a page from the Hy-Line Credit Union in Manitoba:

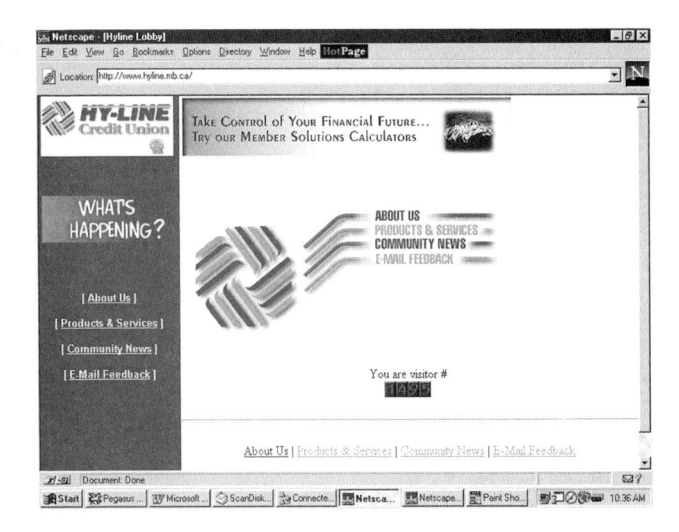

CHAPTER 5 : Cash and Cash-Equivalent Investments on the Internet

Browse through the site, and you'll come across the following section that explains how the credit union protects the deposits of its members:

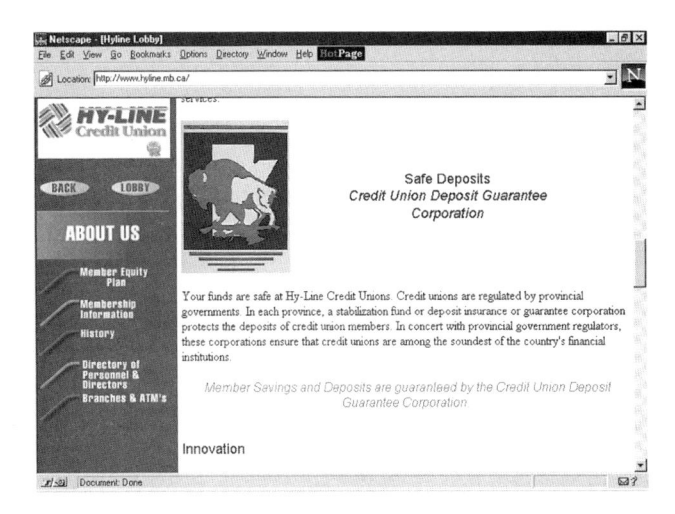

To learn more about the topic of deposit insurance, we recommend you visit the Web site for the Canada Deposit Insurance Corporation (CDIC), which features a concise overview of how the CDIC deposit insurance system works and a list of banks and trust companies that are members of the CDIC. You'll also find a test that you can take to assess your familiarity with the topic.

77

1999 MUTUAL FUNDS AND RRSPs ONLINE

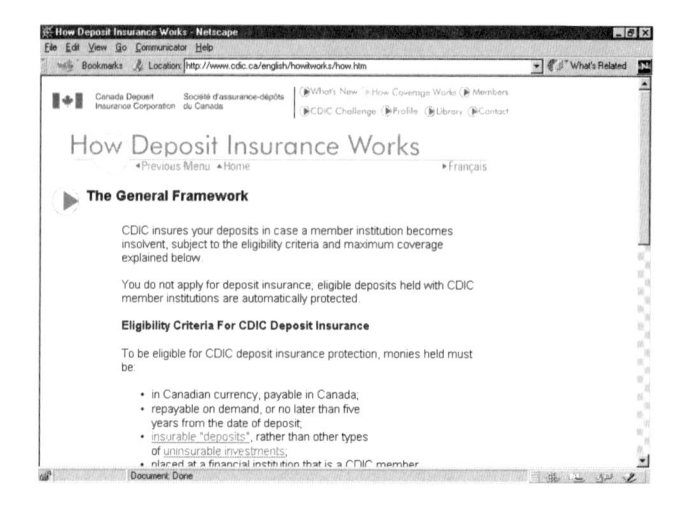

The site also provides helpful information on insurance coverage for deposits held in RRSPs.

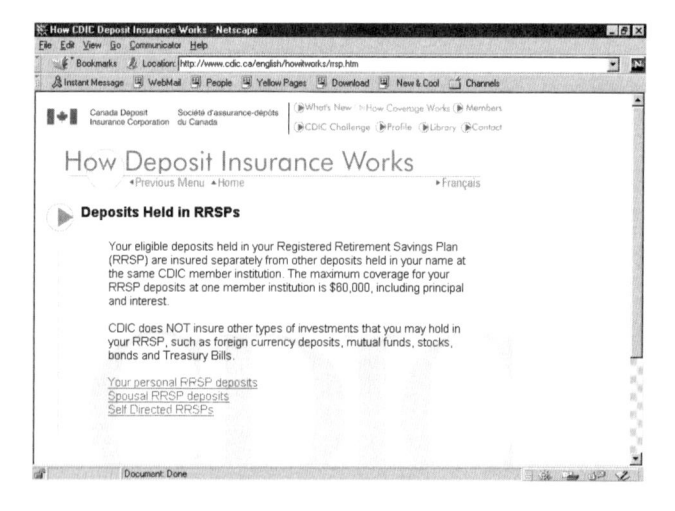

Money held in a credit union is not covered by the CDIC. Instead, it is usually covered by a provincial corporation. Some provincial deposit insurance corporations, such as the Deposit Insurance Corporation of Ontario, have Web sites where you can learn more about the coverage they offer.

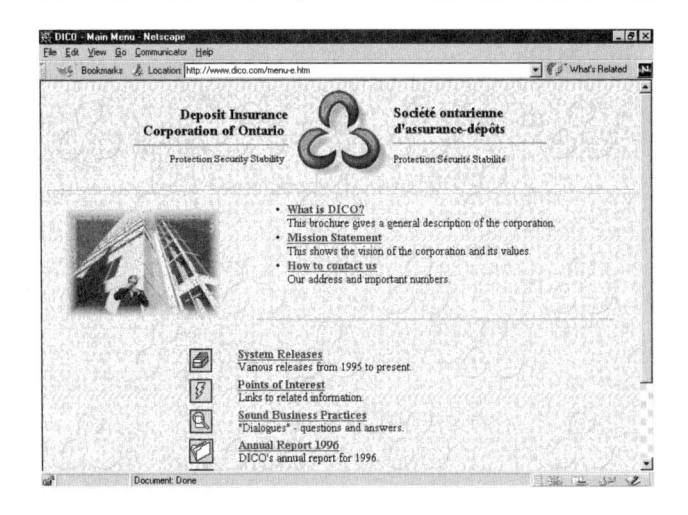

CHAPTER 5: Cash and Cash-Equivalent Investments on the Internet

The Web site for Credit Union Central of Canada, the umbrella organization for all the provincial credit union associations, provides links to most of the provincial credit union Web sites. Visit these sites, and you can usually find out more about the deposit insurance system for credit unions in that province. For example, if you visit the Web site belonging to Credit Union Central Alberta, you will learn that deposits in Alberta credit unions are guaranteed 100%.

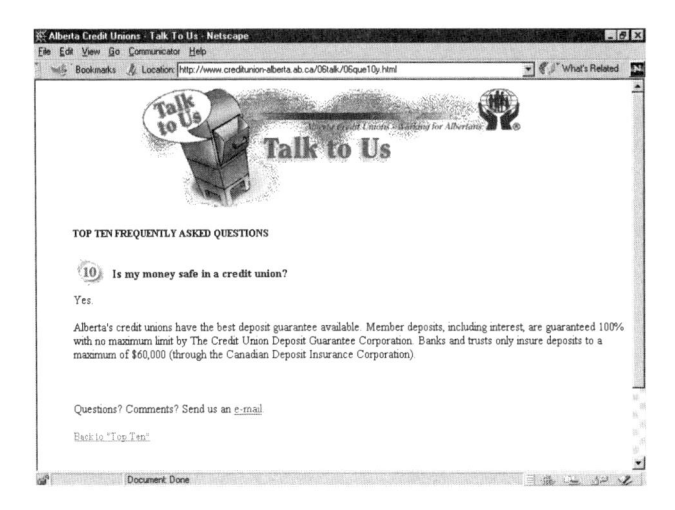

If you decide to place your money in an organization that is not a bank or credit union, you will need to check with them directly to see if they are insured by another organization.

Conclusion

With market volatility, an increasing number of people are turning to cash-based investments. This is where the Internet can play a powerful role, by helping you to quickly compare cash-based investments for the best rates and offerings. Certainly if you invest part of your money in cash-based investments, you'll find the Internet to be a powerful and useful ally in finding the best deal.

Web Sites Mentioned in This Chapter

Canada Deposit Insurance Corporation	www.cdic.ca
CANNEX	www.cannex.com
CANOE	www.canoe.ca
CIBC	www.cibc.com
Credit Union Central Alberta	www.creditunion-alberta.ab.ca/
Credit Union Central of Canada	www.cucentral.ca/
Deposit Insurance Corporation of Ontario	www.dico.com
Hy-Line Credit Union	www.hyline.mb.ca
ilmoney	www.imoney.com
Quicken.ca	www.quicken.ca
Royal Bank of Canada	www.royalbank.com

CHAPTER 6

Mutual Funds on the Internet

Perplexity is the beginning of knowledge. KAHLIL GIBRAN

HIGHLIGHTS

- Most mutual fund companies have Web sites that allow you to obtain descriptions, prices, and other background information about their funds. You can also use the services of sophisticated fund resources such as GLOBEfund, E*Trade Canada (a subscription service), and The Fund Library.

- You can access various tools on the Web that allow you to analyze the performance of various funds or to find the best performers in a particular class of funds. When using these tools, recognize that past performance is not always a good indicator of future performance.

- Online discussion groups can be used to debate and discuss particular funds or investment strategies with other Internet users. Keep in mind that these discussion groups are often used to spread rumours and other misinformation.

If you determine that you want to place part of your retirement (or nonretirement) investment into a variety of mutual funds, you'll quickly discover that the Internet can be a very powerful ally as you try to determine which funds you should invest in.

How can the Internet help you as you wrestle with the issue of mutual funds? In this chapter, we describe some of the ways you can use this technology to help you with your mutual fund decisions. If you are not familiar with the basic mutual fund concepts, we suggest you review appendix C, "Mutual Fund Concepts," and appendix D, "Learning About Investments on the Internet."

Researching Specific Mutual Funds on the Internet

In chapter 3 we outlined the process you should go through to determine what you want to invest in. Our methodology involved using the Internet to understand the various mutual fund asset classes and which specific mutual funds are appropriate for you.

It is no small undertaking to figure out exactly which mutual funds you should purchase. With over 1,800 mutual funds available in Canada, this is not an easy thing to do.

The Internet can both help and hinder you in this regard. The Internet helps, since it makes it very easy for you to obtain individual fund descriptions from most fund companies in Canada. However, the Internet can also be a hindrance because it exposes you to so much information and such a wide array of choices and options. It can be quite overwhelming.

> **Denver-based Janus Mutual Funds (www.janus.com) found that one of the busiest times on their Web sites was at 3 a.m. People were spending that time researching their investments and then calling the next morning to do a deal.**

Once you have identified the asset classes that are appropriate for you, we suggest that you do the following:

- **Compare individual funds in an asset class**
  For example, if you think that at least one-third of your retirement portfolio should be from the equity asset class and that at least half of that should be in aggressive growth funds within that class, examine the various growth funds that are available.

  You can do this by examining mutual fund descriptions at the Web sites of various companies, as well as by reviewing descriptions at all-encompassing mutual fund sites such as The Fund Library, GLOBEfund, and E*Trade Canada.

- **Do a performance analysis**
  Use some of the analysis tools discussed below to identify and analyze the performance of funds in particular categories. This will help you learn more about the track record of particular funds.

These two steps will help you determine which funds you might want to invest in. Let's look at each step in a bit more detail.

Step 1: Compare Individual Funds in an Asset Class—Obtaining Descriptions, Prices, and Objectives of Various Funds

It is easy to access online descriptions of individual funds from the many mutual fund organizations that have Web sites in Canada.

You can obtain a list of the Web sites for most major mutual fund companies in Canada at several of the sites that we have already mentioned, such as The Fund Library, and at the Investment Funds Institute of Canada and the Mutual Fund Switchboard. Or simply visit a Web directory such as Yahoo! Canada and type in the name of the mutual fund company you are looking for.

Keep in mind that while the vast majority of mutual fund companies have Web sites, some companies have been slower than others in learning to market online. As a result, there are still some mutual fund companies without any online presence. Also, among those companies that do have Web sites, some of those sites are more sophisticated than others.

EXCELLENT INTERNET REAL ESTATE

The U.S. company New England Funds was smart to grab the Web address mutualfunds.com. They estimate that a large number of investors who might never have heard of them learn about the company simply by typing www.mutualfunds.com.

What should you be looking for in a mutual fund site? Several things:

- **An overview or description of the fund**
  This would include information about the assets that make up the fund, the risk profile of those assets, an overview of the objectives of the fund, as well as an up-to-date fund management report. Look for details, not marketing fluff. For example, if it is a stock fund, does it actually list the names of the stocks that are held in the fund, or does it just list the types of stocks in the fund?

- **Loads**
  The loads are the commissions that are charged on the fund on purchase (at the front-end) or on sale (at the back-end).

- **Historical performance**
  This information indicates the fund's returns.

- **The management expense ratio (MER) and other expenses charged to the fund**
  The management fee (as an annual percentage of total assets in the fund) and other expenses charged against the fund can be very important factors in the overall return you get on your fund. Take a look at the article "Three things savvy investors are likely to demand," by financial expert Duff Young at the GLOBEfund site. It describes the impact of management fees on your overall return.

- **The background of the investment team**
  What experience does the team involved in managing the fund have?

- **Background information concerning the fund**
  Look for detailed information such as the fund's most recent results, expected outlook, major changes in the fund, and other commentary.

- **The prospectus for the fund**
  Details of the prospectus should be available online, and the site should allow you to request a paper copy. Every fund must have a formal prospectus, which describes the fund in a great degree of detail. Some fund companies place the full prospectus online, while others permit you to easily request a paper copy.

CHAPTER 6: Mutual Funds on the Internet

As we mentioned earlier, you can get information about particular mutual funds from several sources. First, most major mutual fund companies in Canada provide Web sites that contain detailed background information about their particular funds.

For example, Altamira's Web site provides an overview of each of its funds, including background information on the objectives of its funds as well as a listing of the major investments held in each fund.

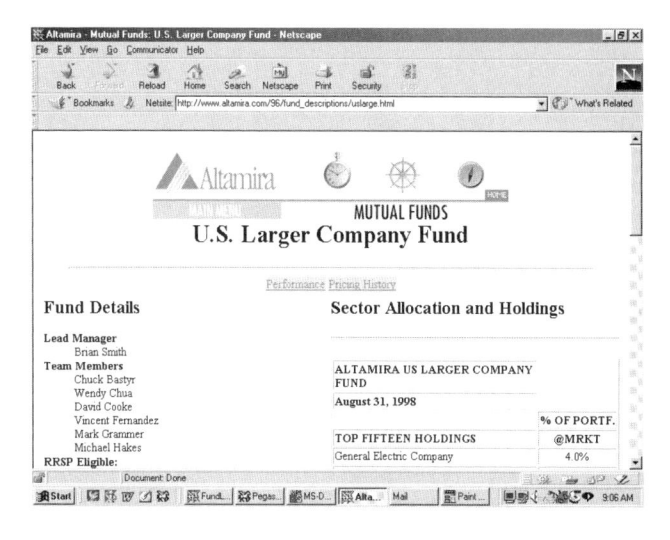

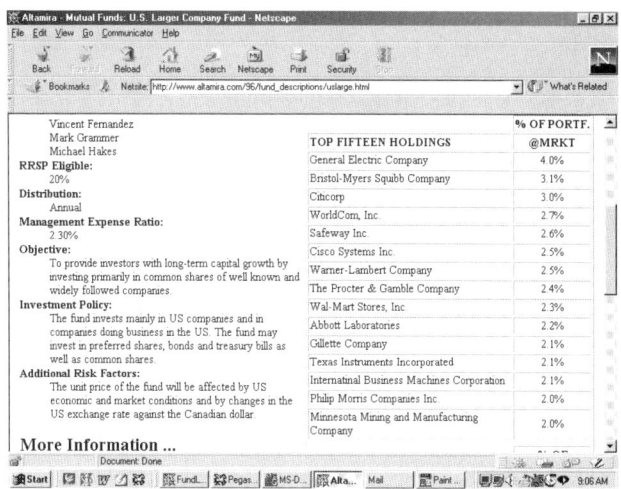

You can also access several sophisticated fund resources that are appearing on the Web. GLOBEfund, an initiative of the *Globe and Mail*, provides access to good, concise

1999 MUTUAL FUNDS AND RRSPs ONLINE

A LIBRARY OF FUNDS

At The Fund Library site (www.fundlibrary.com), you can quickly obtain detailed brochures on a wide variety of Canadian mutual funds in Adobe Acrobat format. This lets you see and print the brochure, exactly as it would have appeared in print. These brochures offer a good synopsis of various mutual funds in a simple, one-page format.

overviews of most Canadian funds. For example, you can access a profile of a mutual fund company:

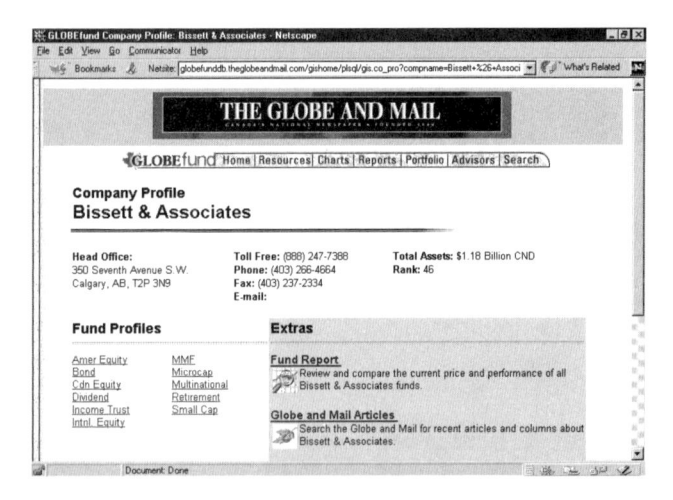

or review details of a particular fund:

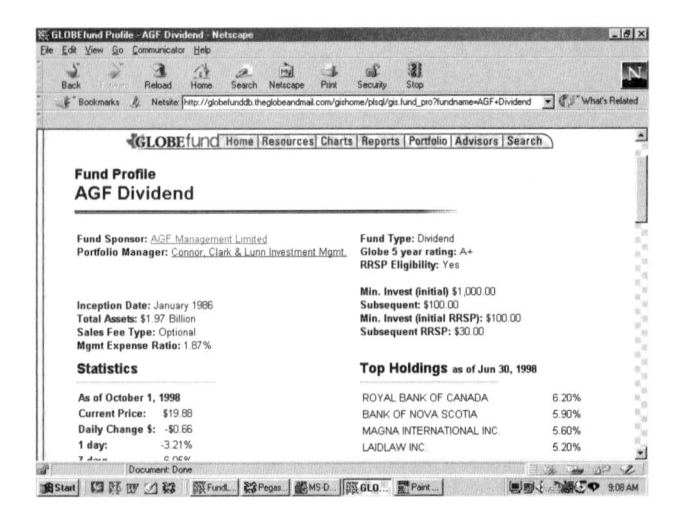

CHAPTER 6 : Mutual Funds on the Internet

The latter includes statistics on the historical performance of the fund, a listing of the major holdings or investments held in the fund, and other information. While looking at a specific fund's Web page on GLOBEfund, you can quickly access news articles that have appeared about the fund, link to the Web site for the fund, or generate a chart that examines the performance of the fund from a variety of different perspectives.

Similarly, if you are a paying customer of the E*Trade Canada online stock trading service, you can access a variety of fund descriptions, such as this graph of the investments held in a particular environment mutual fund:

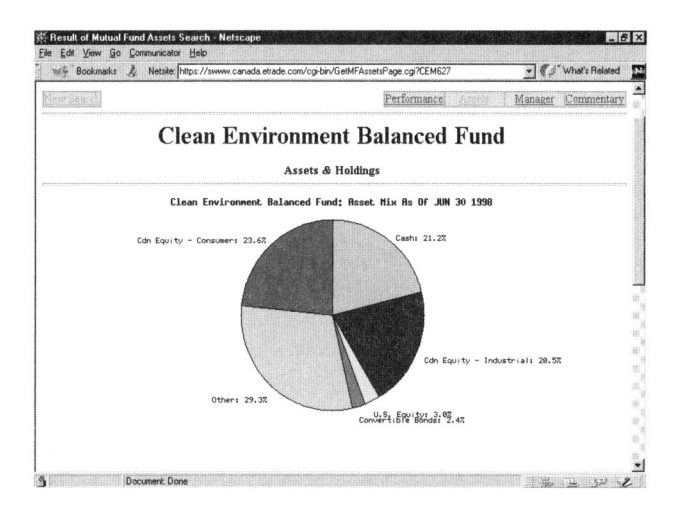

![Screenshot of Clean Environment Balanced Fund Assets & Holdings pie chart showing: Cdn Equity - Consumer: 23.6%, Cash: 21.2%, Cdn Equity - Industrial: 20.5%, U.S. Equity: 3.0%, Convertible Bonds: 2.4%, Other: 29.3%]

You can also use The Fund Library Web site to research Canadian mutual funds; the site provides access to background information on a wide variety of funds. For each fund you can quickly obtain opinions from various Canadian mutual fund experts.

> **One of the best sources to undertake research on a particular mutual fund is the GLOBEfund site (www.globefund.com). It contains several years' worth of articles related to mutual funds and investing.**

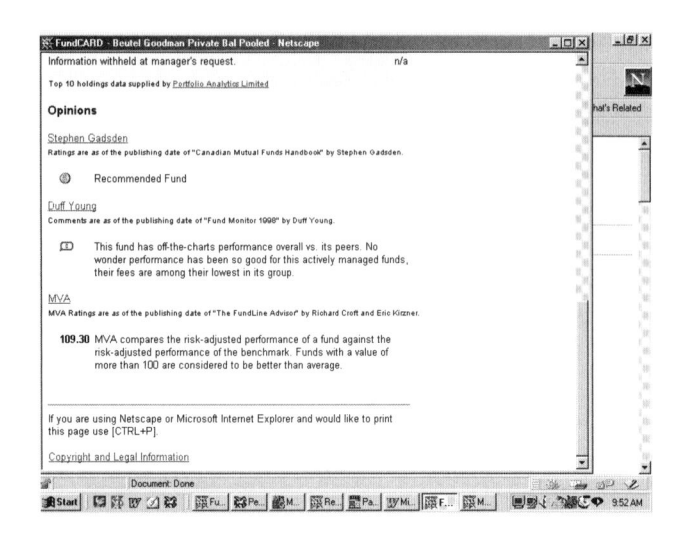

Step 2: Performance Analysis

The physicist Niels Bohr once observed that making a prediction is very difficult, especially when it concerns the future. He might have been talking about mutual funds—particularly when you are trying to use the past performance of a fund to predict its performance in the future.

When looking at various mutual funds, many people look at historical performance information to help them figure out which mutual fund to purchase. Some people believe that the past performance of a fund is a good indication of how the fund will perform in the future. In this line of thinking, identifying the top performers in a class of funds, such as the best performer in Canadian equity funds, can be a useful exercise in getting started or to back up your findings.

Historical performance should not be used as the *only* indicator of expected future performance. Certainly with the market downturn experienced in 1998, historical performance indicators are probably way out of whack with the current potential of many funds.

But if you do want to use performance data to help you decide which funds to invest in, this is one area where you definitely want to take advantage of the Internet. The Internet is full of tools and information that help you examine the performance of a single fund or compare one fund's performance against another.

ONLINE FUND RANKING

To get an up-to-date ranking of mutual fund companies in Canada, visit the Web site for the Investment Funds Institute of Canada (www.ific.ca). In its Statistics section, you can find a monthly report that features a regularly updated ranking of mutual fund companies.

A good place to start is Fundata Canada, a company that supplies daily fund information to the Canadian financial industry. It features a page with the best and worst Canadian mutual funds for the last month, last three months, and the previous one, three, and five years. It's a good place to go to learn about the winners and losers.

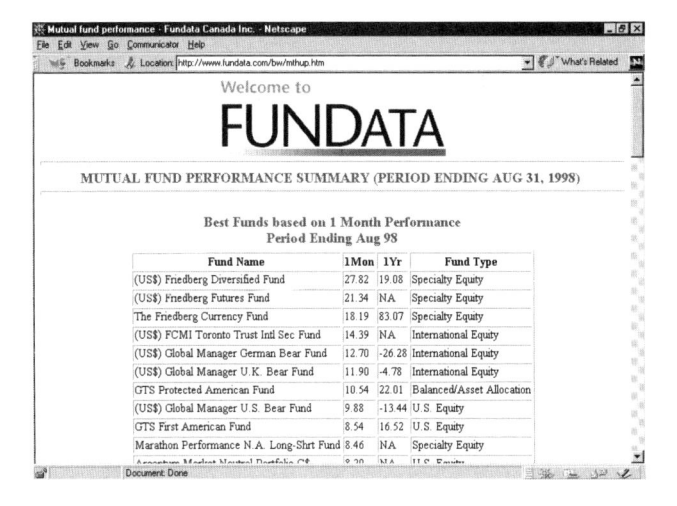

Welcome to
FUNDATA

MUTUAL FUND PERFORMANCE SUMMARY (PERIOD ENDING AUG 31, 1998)

Best Funds based on 1 Month Performance
Period Ending Aug 98

Fund Name	1Mon	1Yr	Fund Type
(US$) Friedberg Diversified Fund	27.82	19.08	Specialty Equity
(US$) Friedberg Futures Fund	21.34	NA	Specialty Equity
The Friedberg Currency Fund	18.19	83.07	Specialty Equity
(US$) FCMI Toronto Trust Intl Sec Fund	14.39	NA	International Equity
(US$) Global Manager German Bear Fund	12.70	-26.28	International Equity
(US$) Global Manager U.K. Bear Fund	11.90	-4.78	International Equity
GTS Protected American Fund	10.54	22.01	Balanced/Asset Allocation
(US$) Global Manager U.S. Bear Fund	9.88	-13.44	U.S. Equity
GTS First American Fund	8.54	16.52	U.S. Equity
Marathon Performance N.A. Long-Shrt Fund	8.46	NA	Specialty Equity

Such rankings of the "best" and "worst" are found throughout the Internet. In particular, check out the mutual fund/investment sections on the Web sites of CANOE, *The Vancouver Sun*, and Bell Charts.

As mentioned earlier, you can use the Web to discover the best performers within a specific category. For example, at E*Trade Canada, a subscription service, you can specify that you want a list of all Canadian equity funds that have exceeded a 2% return in the last month.

1999 MUTUAL FUNDS AND RRSPs ONLINE

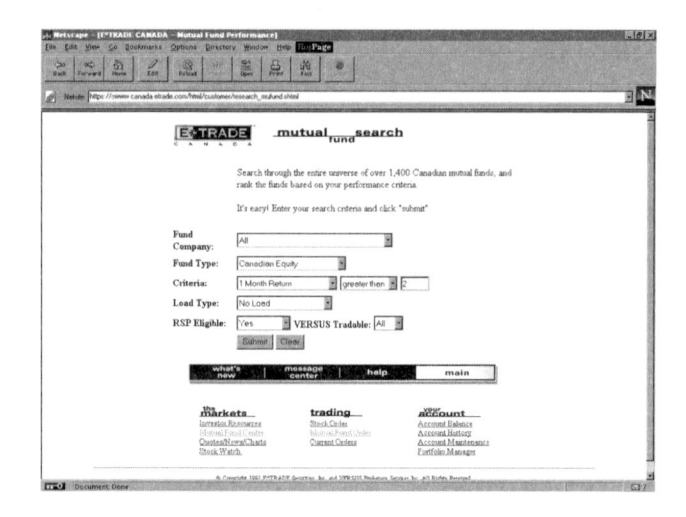

E*Trade Canada then displays the funds that meet the criteria you specified.

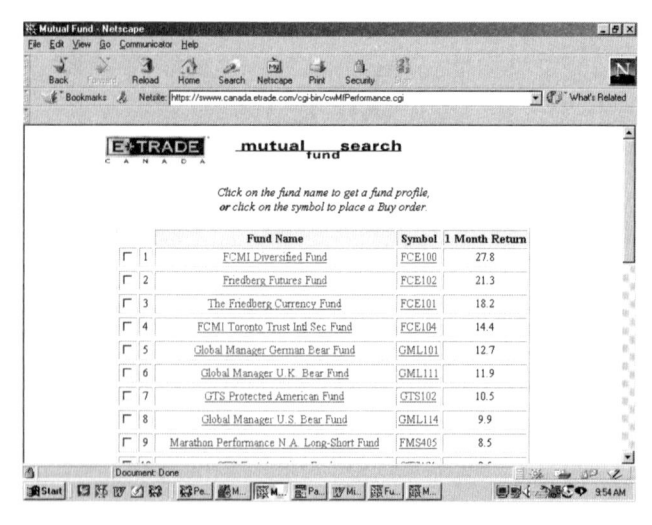

This type of tool can be extremely powerful. For example, if you decide that you want 30% of your portfolio to be equity funds, you can use a Web site such as this one to find the best performers in this category. You can then research the funds on the list to find out which ones are best suited to your needs. To find other performance listings and analysis tools, start out at the Mutual Fund Switchboard site that we mentioned earlier in the chapter.

Finally, GLOBEfund lets you quickly prepare charts examining the performance of a fund against a variety of criteria. For example, on the following screen we've charted the performance of a fund that invests in Asian and Pacific Rim securities against the performance of major companies on the Toronto Stock Exchange (TSE). The resulting graph tells us whether this investment has performed well compared to other potential funds, such as a fund that consists of investments in companies on the TSE.

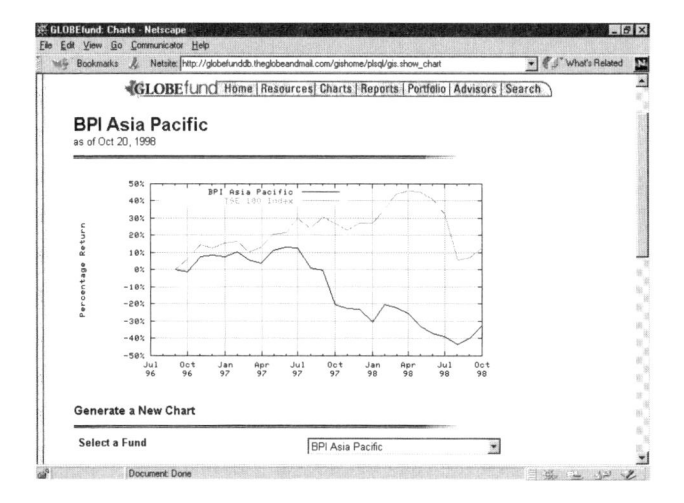

Tools such as these are useful to help you identify potential candidates for your money, but we must stress again that they should not be the only criteria that you use to select your funds. Remember—past performance is not always indicative of future performance!

Online Discussion Forums

Finally, if you are brave and have the time, fortitude, and wherewithal, you might consider visiting a couple of the many mutual fund forums that exist on the Internet, to examine what others are saying about particular fund investments.

> **Want to find other books about investing in mutual funds? You'll find an online library of various mutual fund books at The Fund Library Web site (www.fundlibrary.com).**

1999 MUTUAL FUNDS AND RRSPs ONLINE

For example, at Duff Young's TopFunds site, you can join a number of different online discussions about particular mutual funds:

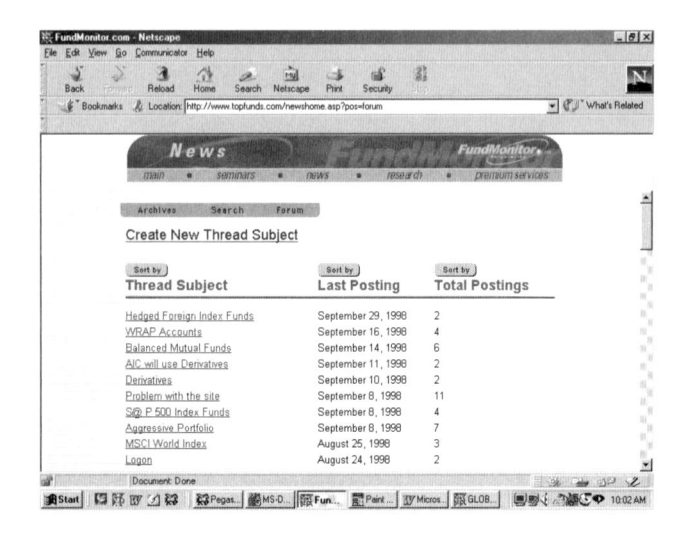

Thread Subject	Last Posting	Total Postings
Hedged Foreign Index Funds	September 29, 1998	2
WRAP Accounts	September 16, 1998	4
Balanced Mutual Funds	September 14, 1998	6
AIC will use Derivatives	September 11, 1998	2
Derivatives	September 10, 1998	2
Problem with the site	September 8, 1998	11
S&P 500 Index Funds	September 8, 1998	4
Aggressive Portfolio	September 8, 1998	7
MSCI World Index	August 25, 1998	3
Logon	August 24, 1998	2

And over at The Fund Library, you can browse through a number of discussions about fund investing:

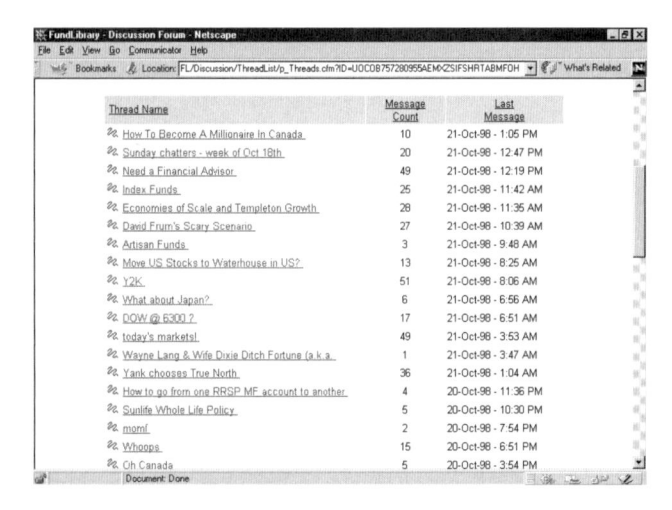

Thread Name	Message Count	Last Message
How To Become A Millionaire In Canada	10	21-Oct-98 - 1:05 PM
Sunday chatters - week of Oct 18th	20	21-Oct-98 - 12:47 PM
Need a Financial Advisor	49	21-Oct-98 - 12:19 PM
Index Funds	25	21-Oct-98 - 11:42 AM
Economies of Scale and Templeton Growth	28	21-Oct-98 - 11:35 AM
David Frum's Scary Scenario	27	21-Oct-98 - 10:39 AM
Artisan Funds	3	21-Oct-98 - 9:48 AM
Move US Stocks to Waterhouse in US?	13	21-Oct-98 - 8:25 AM
Y2K	51	21-Oct-98 - 8:06 AM
What about Japan?	6	21-Oct-98 - 6:56 AM
DOW @ 6300 ?	17	21-Oct-98 - 6:51 AM
today's markets!	49	21-Oct-98 - 3:53 AM
Wayne Lang & Wife Dixie Ditch Fortune (a.k.a.	1	21-Oct-98 - 3:47 AM
Yank chooses True North	36	21-Oct-98 - 1:04 AM
How to go from one RRSP MF account to another	4	20-Oct-98 - 11:36 PM
Sunlife Whole Life Policy	5	20-Oct-98 - 10:30 PM
mom!	2	20-Oct-98 - 7:54 PM
Whoops	15	20-Oct-98 - 6:51 PM
Oh Canada	5	20-Oct-98 - 3:54 PM

You can find additional discussion forums through the Mutual Fund Switchboard.

As you use these discussion forums, keep in mind that the information they contain may be wrong, false, misleading, incorrect, or even downright fraudulent.

> Nicholas Negroponte, founder and director of the Media Lab at the Massachusetts Institute of Technology, predicted that the Internet will take over delivery of investment management vehicles like mutual funds, rendering the intermediary, such as a broker or financial planner, obsolete.
>
> CHRISTINE WILLIAMSON, "ICI TALKS UP EDUCATION, EXPECTATIONS," *PENSIONS & INVESTMENTS*, JUNE 9, 1997, V25 N12 P:35

Making a Decision

We certainly think that there is a lot of useful information online to help guide you in your decisions. But keep in mind that as useful as the Internet might be, your foray into the world of mutual funds comes down to one simple basic rule. To succeed, you must select the fund or funds that best match your investment objectives.

The Internet can provide some information and guidance to help with your decisions, but at the end of the day, it will be your judgment, opinion, and perhaps even your gut feelings or the guidance/expertise of your investment advisor that will guide you in what you decide to do.

Web Sites Mentioned in This Chapter

Altamira Investment Services	www.altamira.com
Bell Charts	www.bellcharts.com
CANOE	www.canoe.ca
E*Trade Canada	www.canada.etrade.com
Fundata Canada	www.fundata.com
GLOBEfund	www.globefund.com
Investment Funds Institute of Canada	www.ific.ca
Mutual Funds Switchboard	web.onramp.ca/cadd/723mut.htm
The Fund Library	www.fundlibrary.com
TopFunds	www.topfunds.com
The Vancouver Sun	www.vancouversun.com
Yahoo! Canada	www.yahoo.ca

CHAPTER 7

Researching Stocks and Bonds on the Internet

Money is better than poverty, if only for financial reasons. WOODY ALLEN

HIGHLIGHTS

- "Financial aggregators" are probably one of the best places to start undertaking research on companies that you are thinking of investing in. Other useful sources of information include news archives and securities regulators sites.

- Online resources such as Carlson On-line Services, the Wall Street Research Net, DailyStocks, and StockHouse provide investors with access to news releases, media coverage, stock data, and other financial information on publicly traded companies.

- It's important to balance the information you receive from a company's Web site with independent information from other sources.

There may be two reasons you are interested in investing in stocks or bonds. First, if you wish to invest your RRSP in something other than mutual funds and cash-based securities, you can turn to the stock market and

95

other investments. To do so, you must set up a self-directed RRSP. This is usually as easy as filling out a few forms at your bank or setting it up with one of the online trading services that we discuss later in this book. Second, you might want to invest in stocks or bonds outside of your RRSP.

In this chapter we take a look at how you can research companies that are traded on stock markets or that have issued debt in the form of bonds, as well as undertake research into the markets or industries in which they operate.

Using the Internet for Company Research

As an investor in stocks, bonds, or other investments, it is important that you understand how to locate online information about companies, their competitors, and their industries. You need this information to help you decide whether to invest in the stocks or bonds they have issued and to judge the safety or future performance of a stock or bond that you already own.

For example, you may want to obtain background information on a company or industry as well as up-to-date reports on a company's financial activities.

Of course, as we point out throughout this book, obtaining the information is one thing, but the most important step is analyzing it. In this section we offer our advice on where to find online information about companies and industries, but we do not provide guidance on how to analyze that information, a topic that is obviously far beyond the scope of this book.

Finding the Company Online

Suppose that you want to investigate a public company's financial and operating history, understand its markets, competitive challenges, outlook, and opportunities, or update yourself on their recent activities. You will want this information in order to weigh their opportunities for success and income against the risks of failure and loss.

Fortunately, both publicly traded and private companies are quickly moving to establish Web sites for a variety of business purposes, one of which is to provide information to existing and potential investors. Organizations will often include their annual reports, press releases, stock information, and other data on their Web sites, making this a useful starting point in your research.

Therefore, your first step should be to determine if the company in question has a Web site. There are several ways to do this:

- If you have the company's annual report, see if it lists a Web site address; many organizations are now including this information in all their investment materials.

- Try searching for the company's Web site in an Internet directory such as Yahoo! Canada or on a search engine such as AltaVista, Excite, or Lycos.

- Call the company's investor relations department and ask if they have a Web site.

It's important to recognize that a company's Web site—if one exists—is not likely to have answers to all your questions. The only information you will find there is the information that the company has chosen to make available online. Also, keep in mind that the Internet is, for all intents and purposes, a relatively new system. Since many businesses are still actively exploring its role, they may not have established a Web site yet, or the site they do have may not have a lot of useful information on it.

Using the information found on a company's Web site is a good starting point, but it's important that you also seek out independent sources from outside the company. You never want to rely solely on official corporate information as the basis for making an investment decision.

> **According to one estimate, by the middle of 1998 there were 95,000 stock trades made each and every day on the Internet.**

Researching a Company

In order to broaden your research, you should use the Internet to examine:

- news reports

- industry analyses
- market histories
- comments from analysts, and
- other independent sources of information.

How else can you obtain information about a company or its industry? There is no shortage of online sources. Check out the Web sites of competitors, if they exist. In particular, search Yahoo! Canada for information on the industry you are researching.

Financial Aggregators

There are several special investor sites online that are designed to help you find information about public companies. For simplicity we will call them "financial aggregators." They make it easy for you to discover multiple Web sites that provide information about a company, making them an invaluable starting point for your research.

Financial Aggregators

Bonds Online	www.bondsonline.com
Carlson On-line Services	www.carlsononline.com
CBS MarketWatch	cbs.marketwatch.com
CNNfn	www.cnnfn.com
Corporate Information	www.corporateinformation.com
Daily Stocks	www.dailystocks.com
Hoover's Online	www.hoovers.com
Integra Information	www.integrainfo.com
Investext Research Bank Web	www.investext.com
invest-o-rama	www.investorama.com
INVESTools	www.investools.com
Market Guide	www.marketguide.com
Multex Investor Network	www.multexinvestor.com
researchmag.com	www.researchmag.com

CHAPTER 7: Researching Stocks and Bonds on the Internet

Reuters MoneyNet.com	www.moneynet.com
SmartMoney.com	www.smartmoney.com
Standard & Poor's Personal Wealth	www.personalwealth.com
StockHouse	www.stockhouse.com
Stock Smart Pro	www.stocksmartpro.com
Wall Street Research Net	www.wsrn.com

A good example is Carlson On-line Services, which bills itself as "the source for Canadian public company investor information and research." Carlson provides quick access to news releases, stock information, and industry data on hundreds of Canadian companies.

For example, suppose you are looking for information about the Canadian mining company Inco. If you do a search for "Inco" on Carlson's Web site, you can access a page of information that includes the latest Inco press releases, contact information for the company, a link to Inco's Web site, research reports, stock charts, and information on the mining industry from Industry Canada. You can also connect to an online discussion group about the company.

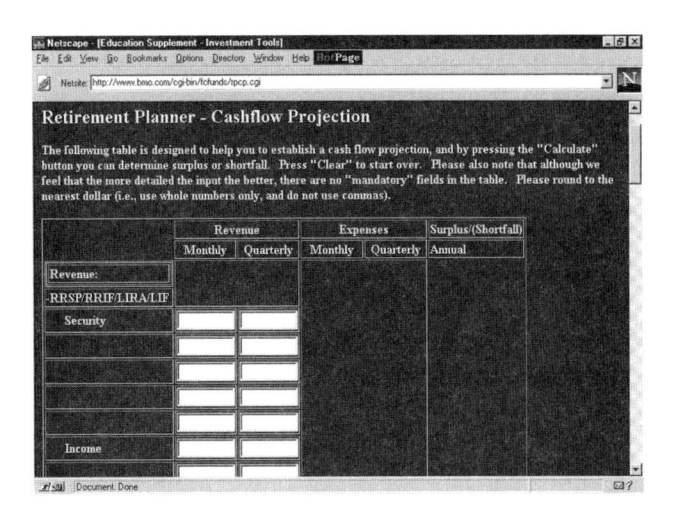

To do the same type of thing with American companies, start out at a site such as invest-o-rama:

99

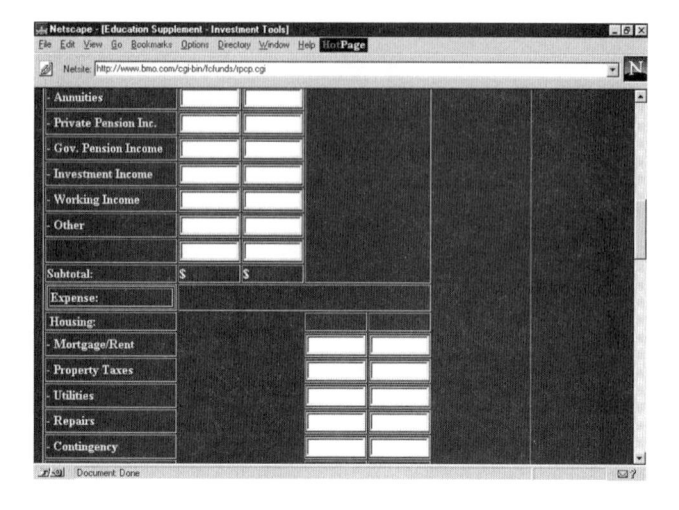

Despite the odd-sounding name, invest-o-rama is an extremely useful site. You can use it to access company information from many different sources on the Internet. Simply type in a stock name or symbol, for example, and you'll get a Web page that features over seventy-five different sources of information about the company.

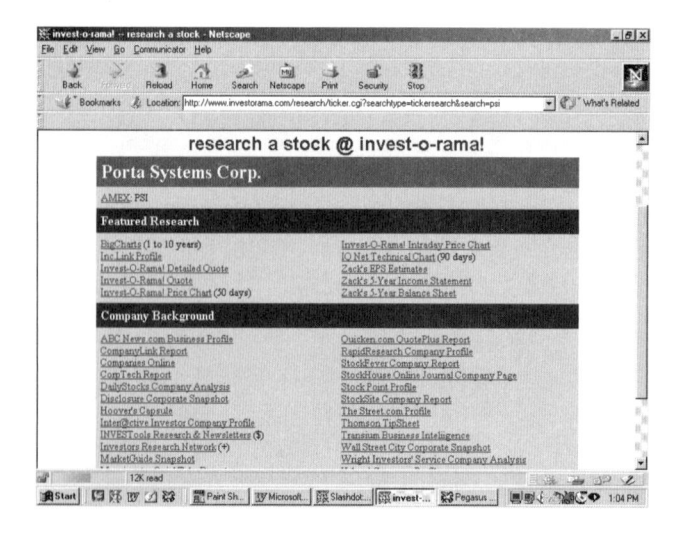

In effect, invest-o-rama has prepared a comprehensive summary of Web sites that include information about the company. Using invest-o-rama, we can retrieve online profiles about the company, stock prices and charts, the filings the company has made with the Securities and Exchange Commission, as well as recent news and press releases.

CHAPTER 7 : Researching Stocks and Bonds on the Internet

If you're researching publicly traded U.S. companies, another excellent starting point is the Wall Street Research Net:

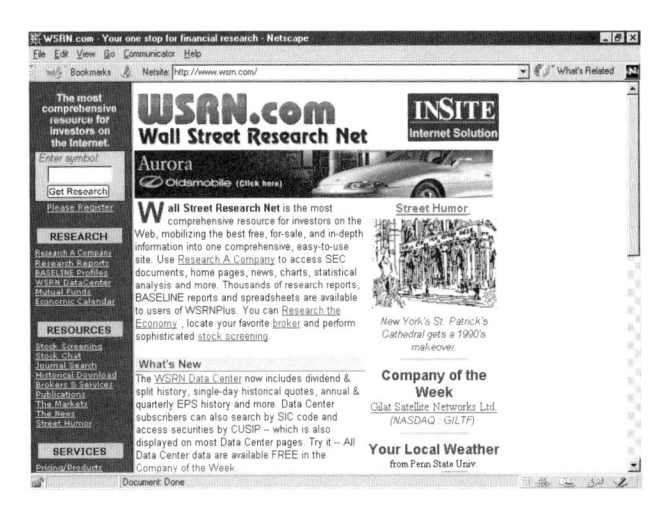

On this site you can access information for over 17,000 companies, including SEC filings, company home pages, annual reports, news releases, stock quotes, graphs, and more. Wall Street Research Net also provides access to economic databases, market news, research publications, as well as links to online brokerage firms, online quote services, and other financial resources on the Web.

Also check out the Daily Stocks Web site, where you can access an incredible array of information about Canadian and American public companies:

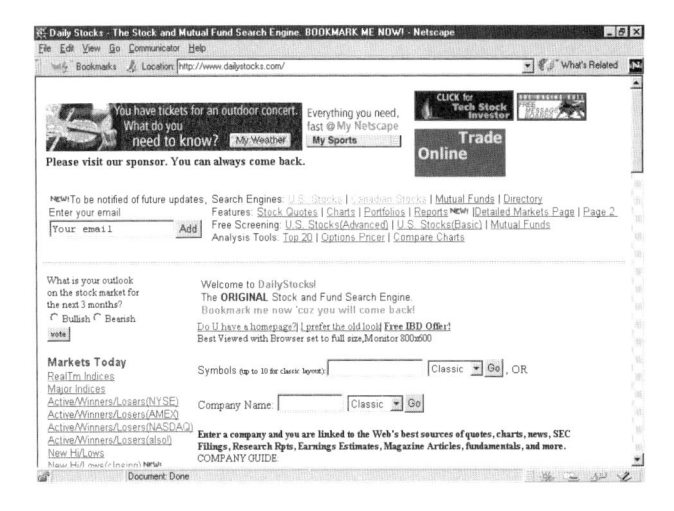

Other popular sites are INVESTools, researchmag.com, and StockHouse.

At StockHouse, you can retrieve press releases for companies; you can also link to news stories that have appeared in major newspapers. For example, in the screen below StockHouse is displaying news items about Suncor Energy that have appeared in the *Calgary Herald* and *The Financial Post*.

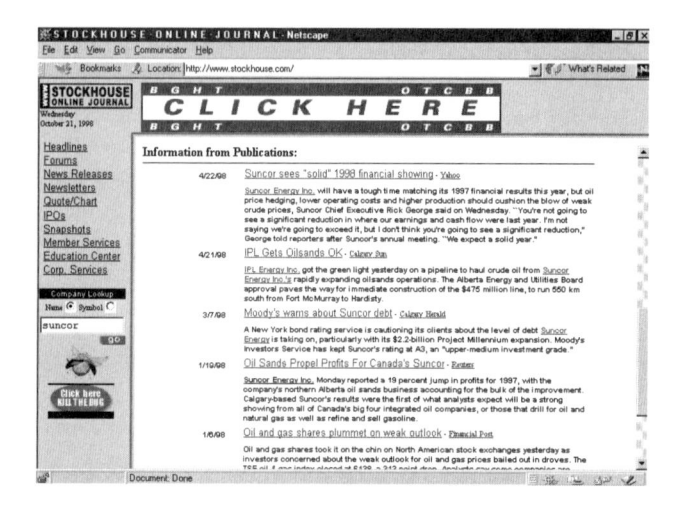

Some of these financial aggregators allow you to conduct research not just on particular companies, but on the industries and markets in which they operate. Many of the financial aggregators are free, but some require you to set up an account to use them. A few charge for the comprehensive industry and market research reports that they make available.

> **It is expected that the growth of systems like the Internet will mean that most major companies will, by some point in the 21st century, trade 24 hours a day on most major stock brokerages around the world.**

News Archives

Many of the financial aggregators listed above will link you to all kinds of up-to-date news information sources, making it very easy to access current data about a company. However, if you are thinking about investing in a certain company, you might want to look into their past as well.

This means that you want to find newspaper and magazine archives.

There are a few places online where you can access such information, some of which are services that charge a monthly fee, others require payment for each document that you wish to read, while some are free. The challenge is knowing where to look.

There actually aren't too many places that you can go on the Internet to access old news stories for free. Newspapers and magazines have quickly come to realize that their archives contain a lot of valuable information; hence many are making the archives available only on a for-fee basis.

However, if you poke around, you can find a few useful locations. For Canadian news archives, start out at JournalismNet, which is probably the best place to find Canadian magazines and newspapers. You can also try the Canadian Magazine Publishers Association Web site, which includes details and links to the Web sites of member organizations, and CANOE, which includes archives from *The Financial Post* and a few other newspapers. You can do a search of news that has appeared within the last 90 days or so, and in some cases longer.

For other newspapers it is pretty well a hit-and-miss scenario: some archive older stories online, while many others do not.

For U.S. news archives there are several places to look. First, visit Pathfinder. Through this site, which was still free when we visited it (although that could change), you can search the full text of many major business magazines in the Time-Warner empire, including *Money, Inc., Fortune,* and others, making this an excellent starting point for research on particular companies.

For example, you can do a search for any articles that appeared in *Fortune* (see page 104).

1999 MUTUAL FUNDS AND RASPs ONLINE

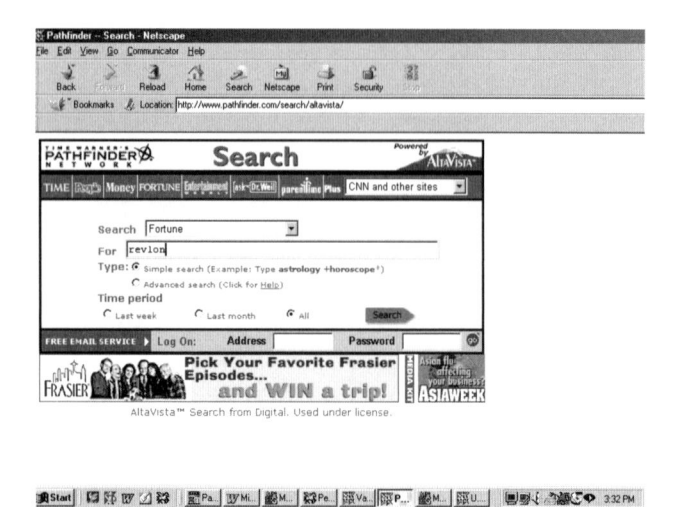

From the list of results you can find news stories from as far back as a few years ago.

With the exception of CANOE, all of these news services have a U.S. focus, but that doesn't diminish the usefulness of their market and company information. Having said that, when you are visiting investment sites on the Internet, it's important that you always check to see whether the service is Canadian or American.

You should also consult online press release services such as Canada NewsWire, Canadian Corporate News, PR Newswire, and Business Wire. Many of these services permit a limited search for past press releases by using a keyword or company name.

If you really want to do historical research into certain companies, there are a number of pay-per-use news archives that provide access to a wealth of corporate and industry information. They are worth exploring for the serious investor.

Pay-Per-Use Services

| Electric Library Canada | Flat fee pricing, with no additional charge per article, of $89.95 per year or $12.95 per month. | www.elibrary.ca |

Encarta Online Library	Flat fee pricing, with no additional charge per article, of U.S. $9.95 per month or U.S. $59.95 for 6 months.	www.iac-on-encarta.com
NewScan	Three levels of membership, each with a different monthly charge and a different per-article charge.	www.newscan.ca
The Wall Street Journal Interactive Edition	Flat fee pricing, U.S. $59 per year.	www.wsj.com
Northern Light Search	Two pricing options: the Subscription offer is U.S. $4.95 per month and includes access to up to 50 articles per month from approximately 1,600 publications. Articles not covered by the Subscription offer are available for U.S. $1 to $4. The second option is Pay As You Go: pay only for what you retrieve, U.S. $1 to $4.	www.northernlight.com
NewsLibrary	Charge for each complete article viewed. Price depends on news source.	www.newslibrary.com

Financial Search Engines

Finally, when undertaking company or market research, you might find that a search within a general search engine such as AltaVista is far too overwhelming in terms of the volume of information retrieved.

That is why you should take the time to become comfortable with finance-specific search engines.

Finance-Specific Search Engines

Alexander Personal Finance Search	alexander.northernlight.com
FinanceWise	www.financewise.com

These search engines index only information that is specifically finance, company, industry or market related. As a result, you can expect better information by utilizing one of these services.

Government Organizations

Various government securities bodies require publicly traded companies to electronically file their regular financial statements and other regulatory filings.

In some cases, this information is then made available to the public through the Internet. A good example is the EDGAR Database (Electronic Data Gathering, Analysis, and Retrieval system), a U.S. Securities and Exchange Commission project. You can search for information provided by various companies on the EDGAR Web site as well as SEDAR, the System for Electronic Document Analysis and Retrieval from the Canadian Depository for Securities.

Online Trading Services

Finally, many of the online stock trading services we discuss in chapter 8 provide access to background information about publicly traded companies. As a result, if you sign up with an online broker, you'll discover a wealth of additional information, some of which might not be available elsewhere on the Web for free.

For example, at E*Trade Canada you can access detailed histories and graphs on particular stocks:

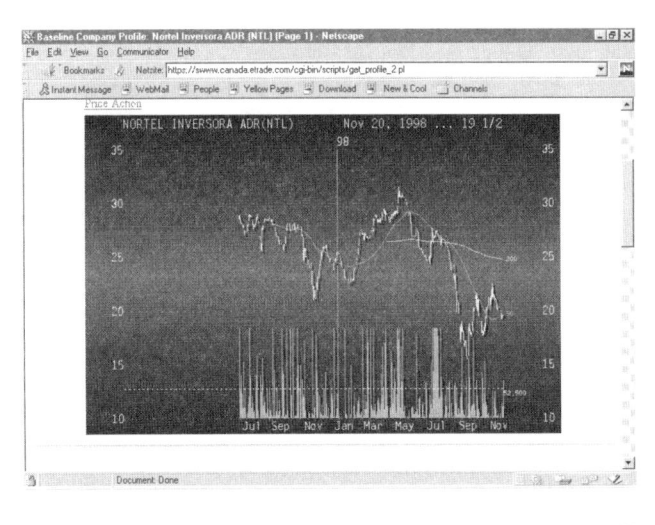

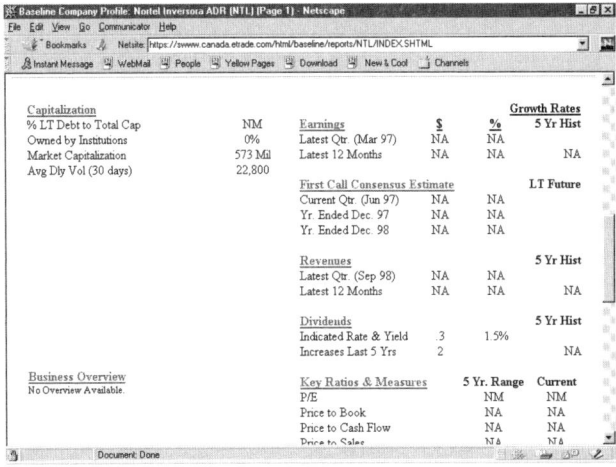

Conclusion

The quality and quantity of information about companies to be found on the Internet is nothing less than truly stunning. As you venture to many of the sites, we believe that you'll be like many Internet users and quickly feel overwhelmed by what you find online.

That is why it is important to concentrate on your original objective: you are here to learn how to use the Internet to assist you in your investment decisions. Hence, carefully assess the information that you find, keeping in mind your original investment goals with respect to risk, growth, and income.

1999 MUTUAL FUNDS AND RRSPs ONLINE

Web Sites Mentioned in This Chapter

Alexander Personal Finance Search	alexander.northernlight.com
AltaVista	www.altavista.com
Bonds Online	www.bondsonline.com
Business Wire	www.businesswire.com
Canada NewsWire	www.newswire.ca
Canadian Corporate News	www.cdn-news.com
Canadian Magazine Publishers Association	www.cmpa.ca
CANOE	www.canoe.ca
Carlson On-line Services	www.carlsononline.com
CBS Market Watch	cbs.marketwatch.com
CNNfn	www.cnnfn.com
Corporate Information	www.corporateinformation.com
Daily Stocks	www.dailystocks.com
EDGAR Database	www.sec.gov/edgarhp.htm
Electric Library Canada	www.elibrary.ca
Encarta Online Library	www.iac-on-encarta.com
Excite	www.excite.com
FinanceWise	www.financewise.com
Hoover's Online	www.hoovers.com
Integra Information	www.integrainfo.com
Investext Research Bank Web	www.investext.com
invest-o-rama	www.investorama.com
INVESTools	www.investools.com
JournalismNet	www.journalismnet.com
Lycos	www.lycos.com
Market Guide	www.marketguide.com
Multex Investor Network	www.multexinvestor.com
NewScan	www.newscan.com
NewsLibrary	www.newslibrary.com
Northern Light Search	www.northernlight.com
Pathfinder	www.pathfinder.com
PR Newswire	www.prnewswire.com
researchmag.com	www.researchmag.com
Reuters MoneyNet.com	www.moneynet.com
SEDAR	www.sedar.com
SmartMoney.com	www.smartmoney.com
Standard & Poor's Personal Wealth	www.personalwealth.com
StockHouse	www.stockhouse.com
Stock Smart Pro	www.stocksmartpro.com
Wall Street Journal Interactive Edition	www.wsj.com
Wall Street Research Net	www.wsrn.com
Yahoo! Canada	www.yahoo.ca

CHAPTER 8

Online Investing

Anybody with money to burn will easily find someone to tend the fire. ANONYMOUS

HIGHLIGHTS

- Many discount brokerages and other firms such as E*Trade Canada offer online trading of stocks, mutual funds, and other investments over the Internet.

- When choosing an online trading service there are many factors that you should consider, including the firm's fee structure and security policy, account features, insurance coverage, and availability of service and support.

- A major benefit of online trading services is that they allow you to trade securities at commissions lower than those charged by full-service brokerages. To compensate for these reduced fees, however, most online trading services do not dispense investment advice.

- The Internet has placed downward pressure on the commissions charged by brokers to execute the sale and purchase of securities. This trend is expected to be especially dramatic within the mutual fund industry.

- To keep yourself up-to-date on developments within the online trading field, you can access the Web sites of online brokers, visit independent news sites, and browse specialized financial sites such as SmartMoney.com.

Now that you've made your way through the complexities of figuring out what you want to invest your money in, the time has come for you to do the actual financial transaction.

If you are investing money in an RRSP and choose not to go the self-directed RRSP route, or if you want to invest some money but you don't want to get involved with the stock market, you will be limiting yourself to cash-based investments and the purchase of mutual funds. In this case, you will likely make your investment by visiting a financial institution or calling a 1-800 number, or you might even purchase an RRSP on a financial institution's Web site.

However, if you opt for a self-directed RRSP, you might consider some of the online investing services that have become available. Similarly, if you are investing money outside of your RRSP, you want to be more involved with your investment decisions, or you wish to buy stocks and bonds, you might consider doing the same.

In Canada today you can sign up with a number of online trading services and buy and sell all kinds of investments through the Internet, including stocks, bonds, mutual funds, and other financial securities.

Discount Brokers on the Internet

Traditionally, if you wanted to buy stocks or bonds, you had to deal with a broker or investment advisor. You would often end up paying a rather hefty commission to buy or sell the investment.

The thinking behind the commission fee was similar to the thinking that exists with load-based mutual funds today—the broker works hard at providing valuable advice and guidance on your investment decisions and, hence, should be compensated for his or her efforts.

As investors began to take on more responsibility for their own investment decisions (for example, by doing their own research), they sought cheaper methods of buying and selling stocks.

The result? The emergence of "discount brokers," organizations that will buy investments on behalf of their clients for a very small fee. In comparison to full-service brokers, discount brokers do not dispense financial advice, and as a result, their commission fees are lower. Discount brokers are popular with sophisticated investors who know what they want and don't require the advice of an investment advisor.

Once the Internet exploded onto the scene, the stage was set for these discount brokers to migrate to the Internet.

> **Online investing systems are not inexpensive. The giant Charles Schwab organization plows some 11% to 14% of its annual revenues into updating its technology so that it remains at the leading edge.**

Today discount brokerages allow you to buy and sell stocks, bonds, mutual funds, and other investments online, either through a Web site or by using a private data network that you can access with your computer.

Researching Internet-Based Online Trading Services

If you begin to explore the field of online investing, there are a number of questions you might have.

Who Offers Online Trading Services?

It is becoming a rather busy marketplace.

All of the major banks in Canada provide online trading/brokerage services through the Internet. In addition, trust companies such as Canada Trust have become involved, as have other Canadian banks such as the Hongkong Bank of Canada.

If you visit the Web sites of Canadian banks and trust companies, you will find information about their online investment services, which usually have their own distinct brand names (for example, netTRADER from the Hongkong Bank of Canada and StockLine from Scotiabank).

> Two U.S.-based research firms, FIND/SVP and Jupiter Communications, indicate that online trading should grow from a current 2% of all transactions to 8% by 2001.

For extremely security-conscious individuals, many of these same institutions offer proprietary software programs that allow you to conduct your transactions through a private data network without going through the Internet. However, the industry seems to have concluded that Internet security concerns are minimal, and we expect these proprietary software programs to become only marginal players in the future.

In addition to the banks and trust companies, other firms have entered the online discount trading market. For example, VERSUS, a private Canadian company that has long served the financial investment community in Canada, teamed up with the U.S.-based E*Trade service to offer E*Trade Canada. E*Trade Canada allows you to trade securities such as stocks and mutual funds over the Internet.

> E*Trade gained notice with the launch of its electronic trading service in 1996, which featured a rather in-your-face advertising campaign. The campaign featured headlines such as "Your broker is now obsolete," "Don't let high commissions bite your assets," and in one ad that featured a kid sticking out his tongue, "Boot your broker."

What Can You Buy and Sell?

Some online trading services allow you to trade only stocks and bonds, while others have added mutual funds to the mix. Those that don't sell mutual funds now will likely do so in the future, simply because of competitive pressure in the marketplace.

Even if an online trading service *does* allow you to trade mutual funds, they might not offer the particular funds you want. Check their Web sites for a catalogue or listing of the funds they allow you to buy and sell.

Interestingly, the field of discount trading often provides some fascinating results. For example, at the TDBank Green Line discount brokerage, you can buy over 800 mutual funds, including those available from the mutual fund subsidiary of the Royal Bank. And at Canada Trust, you can buy funds from the mutual funds subsidiary of the Bank of Montreal.

What About Security?

We don't think that financial institutions would be offering online banking and online stock trading if they didn't believe that their services were secure.

That being said, security should be one of the factors you take into consideration when choosing an online trading service. Most online trading firms provide information about their security measures and policies on their Web sites.

Perhaps the bigger concern is the reliability of the service—there have been reports of people being frustrated by technical problems and challenges with particular online trading services, particularly in the United States.

> **While many online brokerages offered spotty service during a market correction in 1997, most weathered the mid-1998 summer meltdown without any significant service delays or problems. At one brokerage, the time to complete a trade increased from the average of 7 seconds to 16 seconds, which even though a doubling, was a significant improvement over the performance in 1997.**

Is My Investment Insured?

Yes, in the same way that it might be if you had bought it from a broker, agent, or directly from a mutual fund company.

You will find that most online brokers are members of the Canadian Investors Protection Fund, and as a result your investment is covered to a certain maximum amount if the organization where you do your trading collapses.

That being said, you should always keep in mind that you aren't covered for any decrease in the value of your investment due to normal fluctuations in the market.

What Services Are Offered?

Beyond offering the basic capability to buy and sell securities online, some firms provide lots of bells and whistles with their online trading accounts. These services include personalized home pages, e-mail notification if a stock falls below a certain level, access to research reports and company information, 1-800 support lines, real-time stock quotes and news bulletins, and more.

If these "extras" are important to you, make sure that you shop around and compare account features and options. Most online trading services provide this type of information on their Web sites.

What Can I Expect in Terms of Service?

This depends on who you sign up with. Some discount brokers are just that—they will undertake the purchase and sale of securities on your behalf, with no additional assistance offered or provided.

> **No longer associated with techno-geeks, online trading is experiencing a boom in popularity as a growing number of brokerage firms offer it to their customers.**
> RUTH PRINS, "ONLINE TRADING TAKES OFF," US BANKER, MAY 1997

Other discount brokers, such as the Hongkong Bank of Canada netTRADER service, indicate that while they do not provide advice or guidance on which investments to purchase, they do offer a 1-800 number that you can call at any time with other questions that you might have.

Make sure you find out what level of support you can expect before signing up with an online trading service.

What Is Involved in Setting Up an Account?

From the Web site of the Internet brokerage you can either sign up online or you can request that an information package and sign-up form be sent to you.

You will have to deposit sufficient funds with the brokerage to cover your anticipated investment purchases.

You usually do this by sending a cheque in the mail to the online brokerage. In most cases, your account will not be activated until your funds are received. Visit the various online trading Web sites to find out what is involved. At E*Trade Canada, for example, you must deposit a minimum of $1,000.

When you set up your online trading account, you will be asked if the account is to be used for a self-directed RRSP. Some people have several online trading accounts. For example, you might have one for a self-directed RRSP at one online brokerage, and another account at the same brokerage or at another brokerage for other general, non-RRSP investments. Both accounts might hold a mix of mutual funds, cash investments, stocks, bonds, and other financial investments.

What Are the Benefits and Risks of Doing Your Trading Online?

Most organizations that offer online trading services have commission structures that are far less than the commissions charged by full-service brokerage companies. And if you use a discount broker to execute your online trades, the discount broker will usually charge commissions that are even lower than their regular rates because it's cheaper for them to process your orders over the Internet. This means that you're getting a discount on the discount broker's already discounted rates.

Clearly, the primary benefit of using an online trading service is that you can save a lot of money.

In addition, as you get accustomed to doing more of your investment research on the Internet, you'll find that the Internet is a more convenient trading medium.

Why? Suppose you are doing stock research on the Internet and you decide to purchase some shares in a company. Instead of picking up the phone or using a proprietary software program, you simply move from the Web site you are looking at to the Web site for your online trading service, and you can place your order on the spot.

If you are buying or selling a stock that is fluctuating rapidly, the extra few seconds you gain by doing your trading over the Internet could save you a lot of money—but keep in mind that as we pointed out in chapter 2, it is also possible that the Internet will experience a slowdown or technical glitch at the very moment that you are trying to complete your trade. If this happens, the time that you lose could end up costing you a lot of money!

Of course, the cheaper commissions offered by the online trading services come at a price. The trade-off is this: while you will certainly save money by using an online trading service instead of a full-service brokerage, most online trading services don't offer financial advice, and you are responsible for doing your own research.

In other words, you're on your own when it comes to making decisions about which stocks to buy and sell. It's not for everyone.

> **There are almost 100 online brokerages on the Internet.**

Commissions and Fees

When it comes to selecting and using an online brokerage, you should research the fees.

The field of Internet-based investing is causing dramatic change in the investment industry, as increased competition places downward pressure on the commissions charged by brokers for the purchase or sale of securities.

Today, many online brokerages offer a flat fee for stock purchases up to a certain dollar amount. E*Trade Canada, for example, charges a flat rate of $38.88 for most trades or a fee based on stock volume and/or price of the shares you are trading. In the United States, price wars have already broken out among competing brokers. Other brokers have fees that are higher and some have indicated that they refuse to be drawn into a price war.

Of course, all of this makes for a rather interesting marketplace, with constant change in the rates that are charged. The only way to keep up is through news reports and by visiting the Web sites of various online brokers.

Many online brokerage services provide a commission calculator on their Web sites that you can use to determine what commission fee you will have to pay. And as we will see below, you are usually told what the commission will be when you buy or sell your stocks or bonds.

CHAPTER 8 : Online Investing

Browse through the fee schedules offered by major discount brokerages in Canada, and take the time to understand the way their fee structures work. You will find that all of them have a page of information where they describe their fee structure. For example, E*Trade Canada's Web site describes how their transaction fee changes depending on how many shares you are trading:

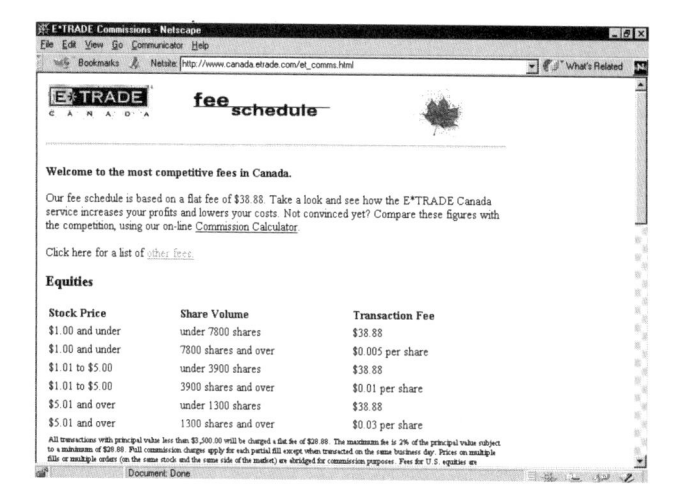

E*TRADE fee schedule

Welcome to the most competitive fees in Canada.

Our fee schedule is based on a flat fee of $38.88. Take a look and see how the E*TRADE Canada service increases your profits and lowers your costs. Not convinced yet? Compare these figures with the competition, using our on-line Commission Calculator.

Click here for a list of other fees.

Equities

Stock Price	Share Volume	Transaction Fee
$1.00 and under	under 7800 shares	$38.88
$1.00 and under	7800 shares and over	$0.005 per share
$1.01 to $5.00	under 3900 shares	$38.88
$1.01 to $5.00	3900 shares and over	$0.01 per share
$5.01 and over	under 1300 shares	$38.88
$5.01 and over	1300 shares and over	$0.03 per share

All transactions with principal value less than $3,500.00 will be charged a flat fee of $28.88. The maximum fee is 2% of the principal value subject to a minimum of $28.88. Full commission charges apply for each partial fill except when transacted on the same business day. Prices on multiple fills or multiple orders (on the same stock and the same side of the market) are abridged for commission purposes. Fees for U.S. equities are

Similarly, at the Toronto Dominion Bank's Green Line WebBroker site, you can access a page that describes their fee structure:

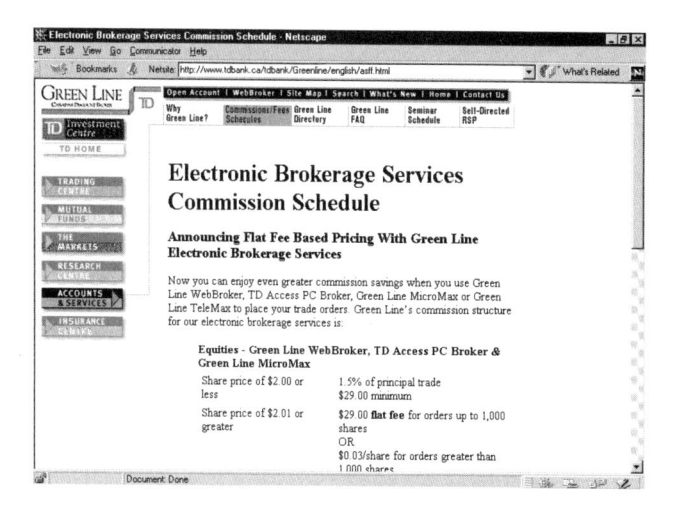

Electronic Brokerage Services Commission Schedule

Announcing Flat Fee Based Pricing With Green Line Electronic Brokerage Services

Now you can enjoy even greater commission savings when you use Green Line WebBroker, TD Access PC Broker, Green Line MicroMax or Green Line TeleMax to place your trade orders. Green Line's commission structure for our electronic brokerage services is:

Equities - Green Line WebBroker, TD Access PC Broker & Green Line MicroMax

Share price of $2.00 or less	1.5% of principal trade $29.00 minimum
Share price of $2.01 or greater	$29.00 **flat fee** for orders up to 1,000 shares OR $0.03/share for orders greater than 1,000 shares

117

Mutual Fund Commissions

The issue of mutual fund commissions bears special attention since it can be a very confusing situation. We suggest that you shop around carefully to understand what your options are when it comes to mutual fund commissions. Keep in mind these two facts:

- Some organizations don't charge any basic trading commission on mutual funds. Others do, based on the type of mutual fund.

- If you are told there is no commission on execution of a mutual fund trade, there isn't—at least, not the $40 or so trading commission described above. Yet the online trading company is still keeping the "load" or commission on the sale of a loaded mutual fund. In effect, it is earning that money as a commission for conducting the sale. Similarly, it might be earning a "trailer fee" once you sell the fund.

Let's have a look at how the situation can vary from company to company.

At the CT Securities Web site, the online home of the investment arm of Canada Trust, you might find that the commission rates on mutual funds vary depending on whether it is a no-load, front-load, or back-load fund (we explain these concepts in appendix C):

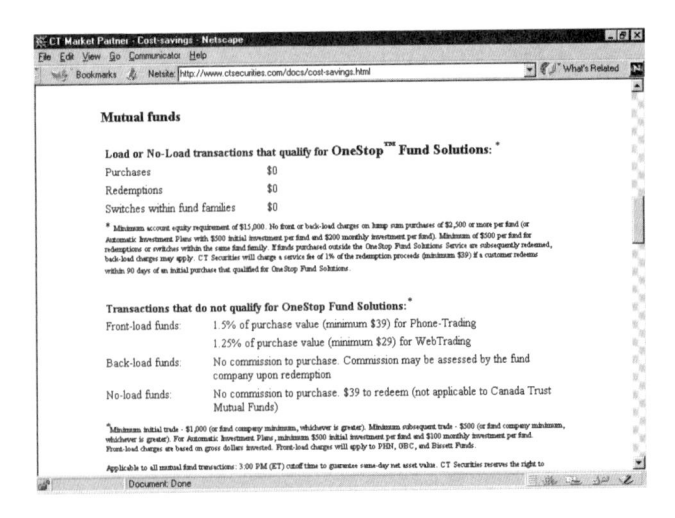

CHAPTER 8 : Online Investing

But at E*Trade Canada, you might find that the commission they charge on most mutual funds is "free," but that there are a few fine print items:

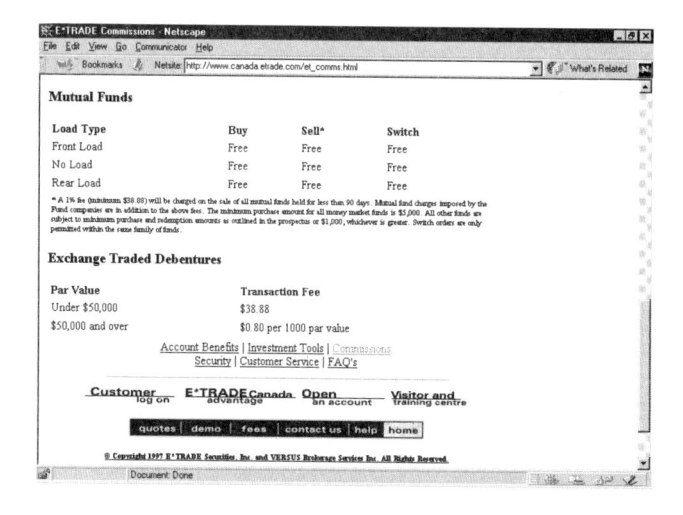

At Scotiabank the fee depends on the type of fund purchased. The fee varies from no fee to a percentage based on the dollar value purchased:

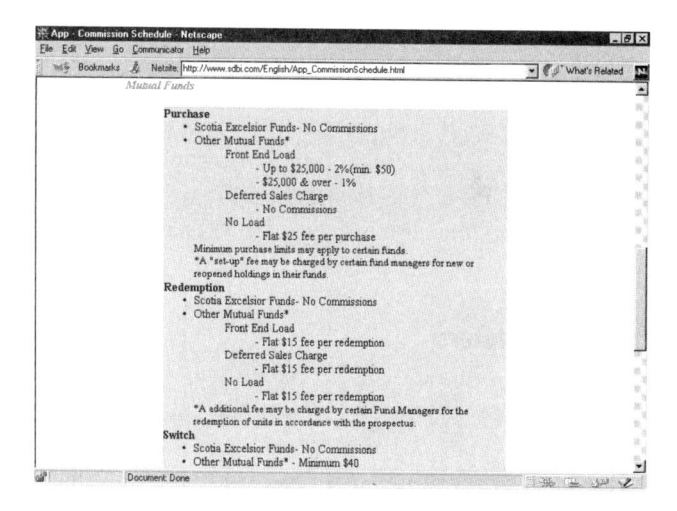

How can some companies buy and sell mutual funds for you and not charge for it? Why do others charge a fee? This is part of the turmoil that exists in the newly emerging field of online mutual fund sales.

119

To understand why things are so different, and why they will, no doubt, keep evolving, you should keep in mind several factors:

- Some online brokers will argue that they charge a fee because they are still providing investment counsel and advice that would previously have been supplied by the financial planner, broker, or agent.

- In many cases, even though you might not be charged a commission, the broker will still be receiving a fee from the mutual fund company. This will come either as a commission up-front (for load funds), on your sale of the fund (as a back-end load), or in the form of a "trailer fee" just as a financial planner or agent would if you bought the funds direct from them. Trailer fees are paid to whoever sold you the fund; the fees are for investment advice on an ongoing basis in addition to front- or back-end loads. All mutual funds charge trailer fees.

Given the current turmoil, it is likely that the entire issue of online mutual fund fees will change with dramatic speed. We discuss this issue further at the end of this chapter.

One other word of advice. When researching the fees on mutual funds, it is important that you study the fine print. For example, you will find that many brokerages will charge a fee if you don't hold a fund for a certain period of time, and sometimes a fee is charged if you move your money from one fund to another.

Online Calculators

Finally, while you're researching commissions, keep your eye out for one very useful feature—the online commission calculator.

Many discount brokerages have calculators on their Web sites that you can use to calculate the commission that you will be charged on a certain trade. This can be useful if the fee is an important factor for you when choosing an online broker. The calculators can help you understand how the commission structures work.

Often a discount broker will compare their fees to those charged by their competitors. For example, at

CHAPTER 8 : Online Investing

E*Trade Canada you can calculate the commission E*Trade Canada would charge on a stock trade. Simply enter the share price and the number of shares you want to purchase:

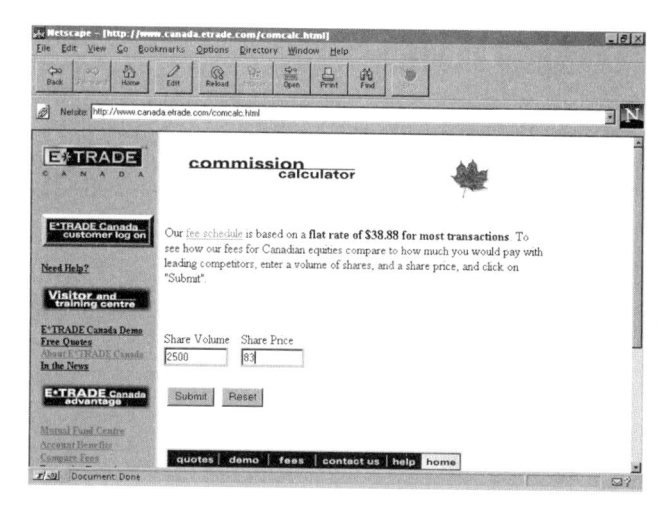

Based on the information you supply, E*Trade Canada will calculate its commission and show you what other discount brokers would charge:

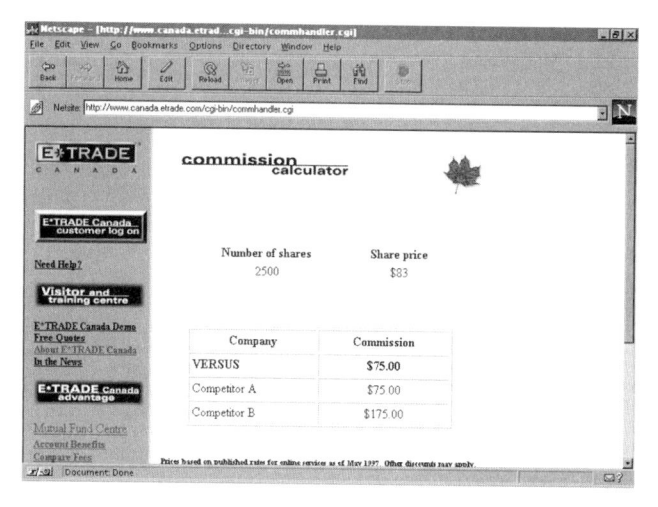

While these calculators are useful, you should be wary of the comparison. Be sure to check that any comparative calculations like this are based on the most recent fee schedules of other discount brokers. If the Web site doesn't tell you which company its fees are being compared to, ask!

121

If in doubt, check the math yourself, or ask the discount broker for confirmation that the calculator reflects the current commission structures of their competitors.

An Example of Online Trading

Once you've signed up with a particular online broker, you will find that the process of buying and selling stocks, bonds, or mutual funds is remarkably straightforward.

> A 1998 survey of online investors by the online financial site thestreet.com found that the investors valued the reliability of the online service over low commissions.

In the hypothetical example below, we'll examine how E*Trade Canada works, and operate under the assumption that you already have an E*Trade Canada account.

Let's say you want to purchase shares in Noranda. First, you fill out the stock purchase form on the E*Trade Canada Web site, indicating the number of shares you would like to purchase. You must indicate whether you are willing to buy at the current market price, whatever it might be, or whether there is a limit on the price you are willing to pay:

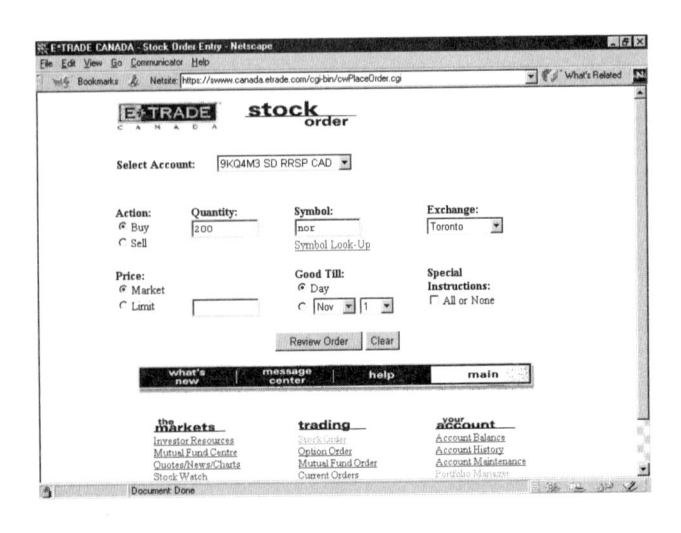

CHAPTER 8 : Online Investing

Once you have entered the details of your order, you'll receive a screen confirming them, which also indicates the commission that will be charged on the order. Obviously, you should review the information on this screen very carefully.

If you want to go ahead with the trade, you provide your "trading password," which is a special password that you will have created strictly for the purpose of confirming your online orders.

> **In an online poll undertaken in October 1998, MSNBC found that 42% of respondents rated their online broker as fair or poor.**

Once your order has been placed, it will be executed by VERSUS Brokerage according to your instructions. After the order has been placed, you can check on its status and modify it if necessary. If it has been executed, you'll be notified.

Of course, if you don't have sufficient funds in your account when you attempt to execute an order, you'll be told:

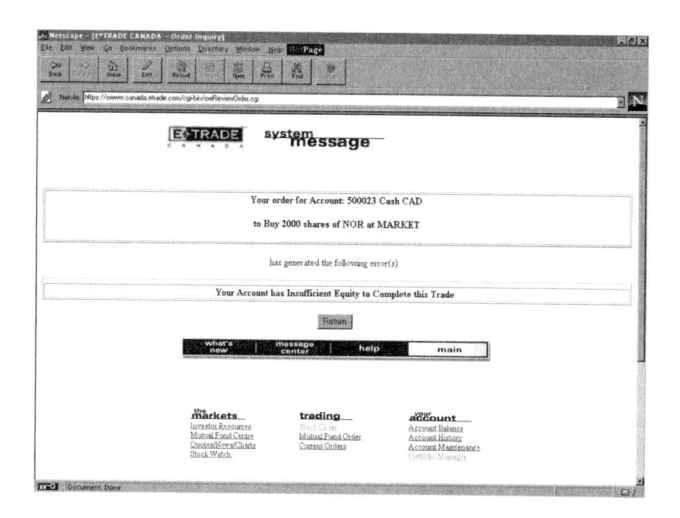

1999 MUTUAL FUNDS AND RRSPs ONLINE

You can review a listing of the cash and securities you have in your E*Trade Canada account at any time:

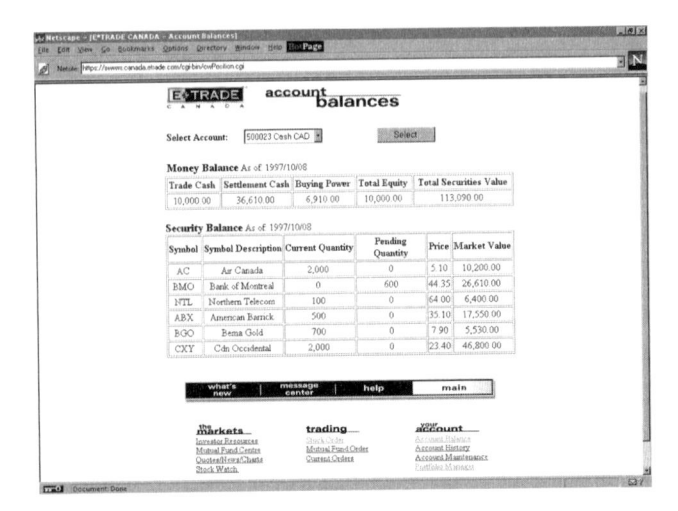

What happens if you want to buy mutual funds? The first thing to keep in mind is that like all other online brokers, E*Trade Canada lets you view a listing of the funds that they allow you to buy and sell:

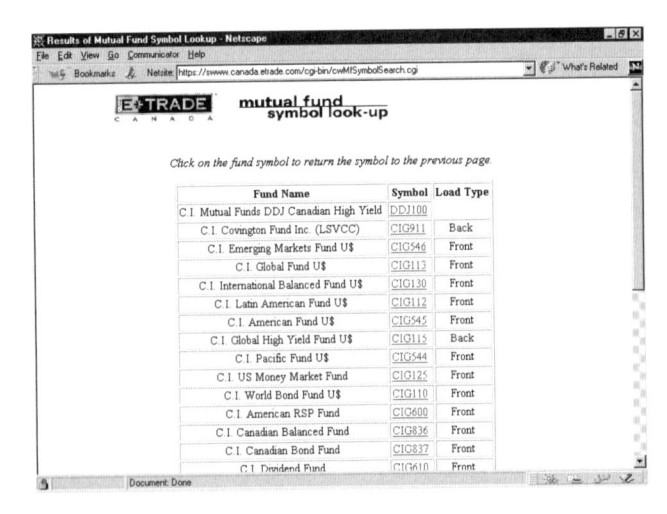

Placing a mutual fund order is no more complicated than buying shares in a stock:

CHAPTER 8 : Online Investing

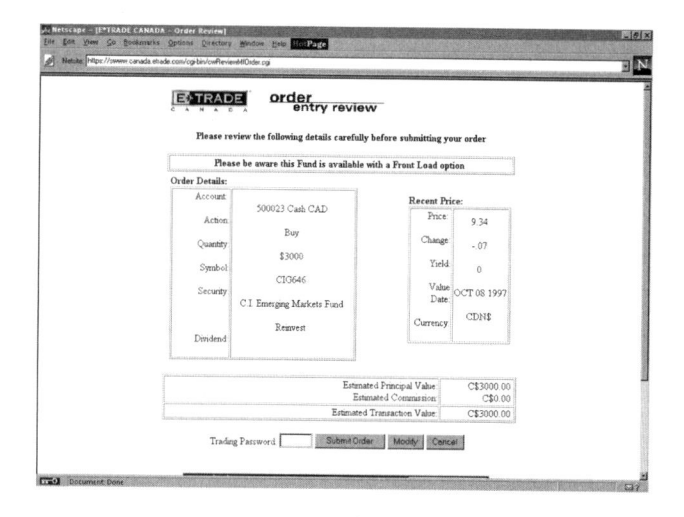

[Screenshot of E*TRADE Canada Order Entry Review page showing order details: Account 500023 Cash CAD, Action Buy, Quantity $3000, Symbol CIG646, Security C I Emerging Markets Fund, Dividend Reinvest; Recent Price: 9.34, Change -.07, Yield 0, Value Date OCT 08 1997, Currency CDN$; Estimated Principal Value C$3000.00, Estimated Commission C$0.00, Estimated Transaction Value C$3000.00]

You go through a similar series of steps if you want to sell stocks, bonds, or mutual funds.

Continuing to Learn About Online Trading

Since this industry is changing so rapidly, it's important to keep up with the changes. The Internet will be very useful to you as you continually assess the features, costs, benefits, and value-added services associated with the various online trading firms.

Web Sites

The most obvious way of gathering information about online trading is to visit the Web sites of the online brokers themselves. In the table below, we've summarized the addresses of some of the major online trading services in Canada.

Web Addresses for Online Trading Services in Canada

Bank of Montreal: InvestorLine	www.investorline.com
CIBC: Investor's Edge Discount Brokerage	www.cibc.com
CT Securities (Canada Trust): Market Partner	www.ctsecurities.com
E*Trade Canada	www.canada.etrade.com

Hongkong Bank of Canada Discount Trading: netTRADER	nettrader.hkbc.ca
InvesNET	www.invesnet.com
Priority Brokerage	www.prioritybrokerage.com
Royal Bank Action Direct	www.royalbank.com
Scotia Discount Brokerage (Scotiabank): StockLine	www.sdbi.com
Toronto Dominion Bank: Green Line WebBroker	www.greenline.ca

By visiting these sites you can obtain information on each firm's commission structure, security policy, range of services, account types, insurance coverage, and more. Use this information to help you decide which online brokerage best meets your needs.

Some online brokers, like Green Line, the discount brokerage arm of the Toronto Dominion Bank, have news sections on their Web sites with information about recent enhancements to their offerings:

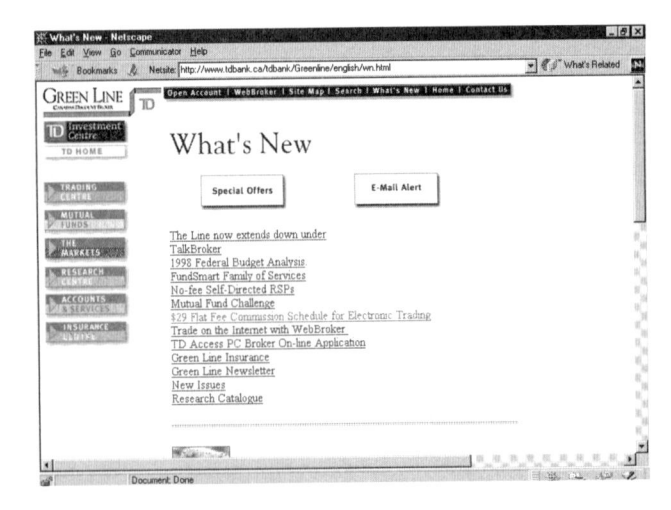

Online News Archives

It's important that you balance any information you receive from the discount brokers with information from an independent source such as a newspaper. On some news sites, you can look at archived news stories and do a search for articles that have referred to online trading in the past few

CHAPTER 8 : Online Investing

months. This is a very useful way to keep on top of the changes that might have occurred within the industry.

Two notable places to visit to obtain this independent verification are CANOE and GLOBEfund.

- **CANOE**

    At this site you can quickly and easily retrieve articles that have appeared in *The Financial Post* during the last several months. From the main CANOE home page, select "Search."

    In the example below, we're looking for any articles that contain the words "Internet" and "trading."

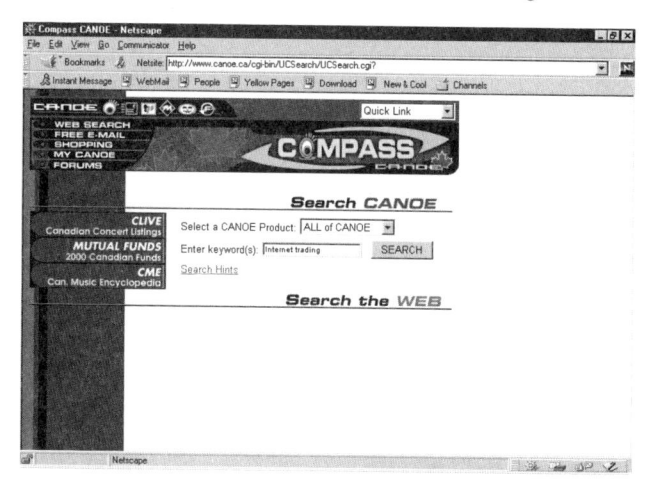

    CANOE searches its database and displays a list of candidate articles. From here, you can access any of the articles shown on the screen without charge:

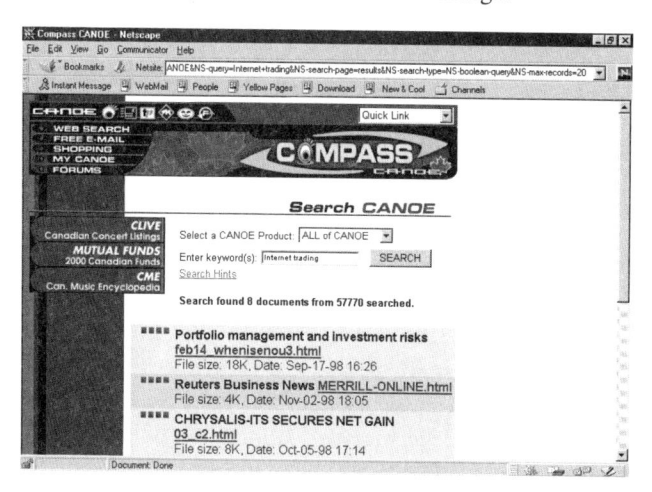

- **GLOBEfund**

    At this site, you can search the full text of articles from the *Globe and Mail*'s special mutual fund reports. Sometimes you can find useful articles about online trading here. Simply key in the phrase you are looking for:

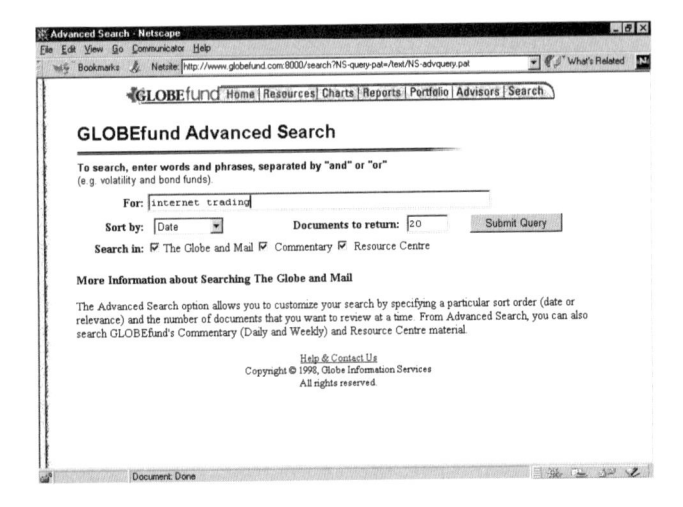

    Next, GLOBEfund will display a list of matching articles:

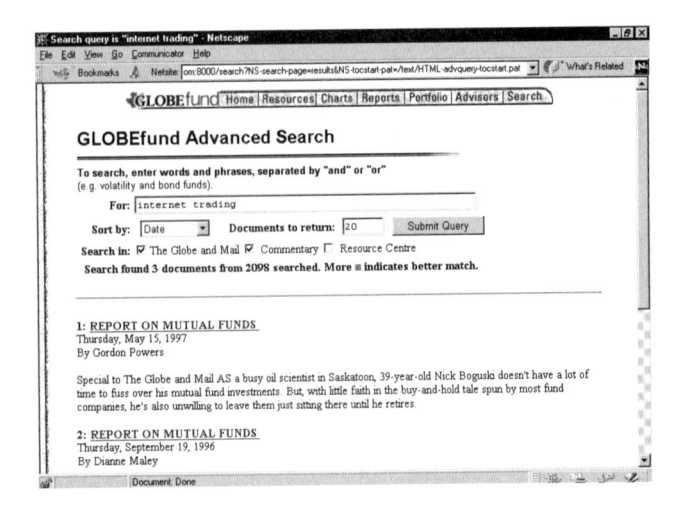

    To access the full text of any of the articles, just click on the headline of the article you want to view.

CHAPTER 8 : Online Investing

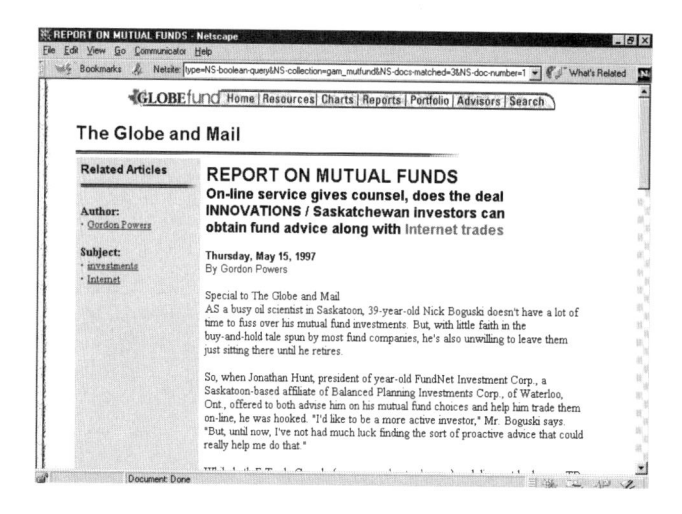

There are also specialized financial news sites such as CNNfn and SmartMoney.com (shown below). Although most of them are U.S.-centric, they can still help you to keep up with recent developments in the industry.

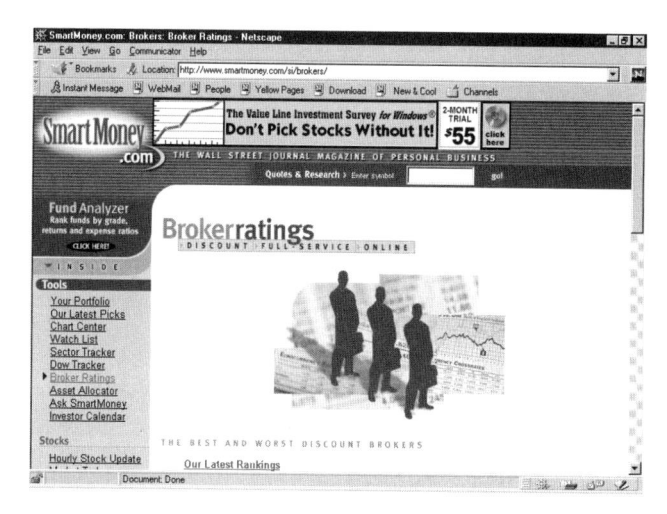

The Future?

What can we expect in the future?

There is no doubt that the entire field of online trading promises to be one that is constantly evolving and rapidly changing.

We have no doubt that more of the major American online stock trading services will enter the marketplace, either through their Canadian subsidiaries or by partnering with an existing Canadian financial institution. For example, American Express is a major player in the U.S. market, as is Charles Schwab with their e.Schwab online trading service.

> **According to Forrester Research, the number of brokerage accounts on the Internet will rise from 3 million in late 1997 to 14.4 million in 2002.**

There are various organizations that track developments in the online brokerage industry. One such organization is Gomez Advisors. One of the items on their Web site is a ranking of the major American online services:

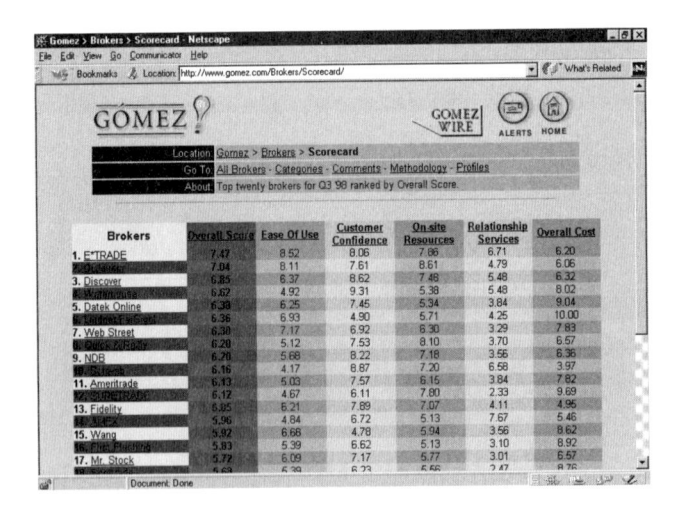

Brokers	Overall Score	Ease Of Use	Customer Confidence	On-site Resources	Relationship Services	Overall Cost
1. E*TRADE	7.47	8.52	8.06	7.86	6.71	6.20
2. Schwab	7.04	8.11	7.61	8.61	4.79	6.06
3. Discover	6.85	6.37	8.62	7.48	5.48	6.32
4. Waterhouse	6.63	4.92	9.31	5.38	5.48	8.02
5. Datek Online	6.38	6.25	7.45	5.34	3.84	9.04
6. DLJdirect	6.36	6.93	4.90	5.71	4.25	10.00
7. Web Street	6.30	7.17	6.92	6.30	3.29	7.83
8. Quick & Reilly	6.20	5.12	7.53	8.10	3.70	6.57
9. NDB	6.20	5.68	8.22	7.18	3.56	8.36
10. Suretrade	6.16	4.17	8.87	7.20	6.58	3.97
11. Ameritrade	6.13	5.03	7.57	6.15	3.84	7.82
12. SURETRADE	6.12	4.67	6.11	7.80	2.33	9.69
13. Fidelity	6.05	6.21	7.89	7.07	4.11	4.96
14. A.B. Watley	5.96	4.84	6.72	5.13	7.67	6.46
15. Wang	5.92	6.68	4.78	5.94	3.56	8.62
16. Bull & Bear	5.83	5.39	6.62	5.13	3.10	8.92
17. Mr. Stock	5.72	6.09	7.17	5.77	3.01	6.57

The second significant change that online trading will lead to is a dramatic change in the load that is charged on various mutual funds in Canada, as more and more sales occur through online brokers. This in itself will lead to significant change in the overall structure of the mutual funds industry in Canada.

Why will the industry change so significantly? The emergence of Internet-based mutual fund sales means that you can now buy "load" (commission-based) mutual funds from a number of online systems. Previously, the companies that sold these mutual funds would have

> **Forrester Research estimates that at least half of Internet-based brokerage services are profitable, and another 20% are break-even, making this one of the few areas of the Internet where companies are actually making money online.**

directed you to a financial planner, broker, or agent to complete the sale. In essence, the commission was built into the fund to provide a return to this third party.

But with the emergence of the Internet, sales of load funds are now occurring through a third party—the online broker—who in most cases is not acting as an investment advisor and often does little to facilitate the sale of the load fund, other than shuffle a few electronic bits. Yet that discount broker is still earning the full "load" on the sale of the load fund to you, in addition to earning a trailer fee.

Hence, while the online discount brokers might state on their Web sites that there is no straight trading commission on the fund, such as the commission of $40 or so that we described above, they are still keeping the load provided to them directly from the mutual fund company. This can often be a substantial sum of money.

We expect that over time, the Internet will drive down the load provided on these types of mutual funds—a significant change for an industry that has been built around the concept of commission-based mutual funds.

Web Sites Mentioned in This Chapter

American Express	www.americanexpress.com/canada/index.html
Bank of Montreal	www.bmo.com
Canada Trust	www.canadatrust.com
Canadian Investor Protection Fund	www.cipf.ca
CANOE	www.canoe.ca
CIBC	www.cibc.com
CNNfn	www.cnnfn.com

CTSecurities	www.ctsecurities.com
e.Schwab (Charles Schwab)	www.eschwab.com
E*Trade Canada	www.canada.etrade.com
GLOBEfund	www.globefund.com
Gomez Advisors	www.gomezadvisors.com
Hongkong Bank of Canada	www.hkbc.ca
InvesNET	www.invesnet.com
Priority Brokerage	www.prioritybrokerage.com
Royal Bank of Canada	www.royalbank.com
Scotiabank	www.scotiabank.ca
SmartMoney.com	www.smartmoney.com
Toronto Dominion Bank	www.tdbank.ca

CHAPTER 9

Monitoring Your Performance

The chief value of money lies in the fact that one lives in a world in which it is overestimated. H. L. MENCKEN

HIGHLIGHTS

- There are many online calculators that you can use to determine the maturity value of a GIC or term deposit.

- You can track the value of your mutual fund holdings on the Internet in four ways: by looking up the daily net asset value of your funds, by generating simple reports and graphs, by using sophisticated "portfolio trackers" such as those offered by The Fund Library and GLOBEfund, and by using portfolio management software such as PALTrak.

- You can obtain delayed and real-time stock quotes on the Internet, many of them for free. QuotesCanada.com is one such free service.

- Using Quicken, sophisticated personal financial management software, you can manage all your investment needs and link to the Internet for current Canadian mutual fund, stock, and other investment data.

After you have made your way through the complexities of figuring out what you want to invest your money in, it is time to monitor the performance of your investments.

Take a deep breath. As you venture further into the world of online finance, you will discover that there are all kinds of methods you can use to track how you are doing.

This chapter examines how you can use the Internet to monitor the performance of your cash-based investments, mutual funds, and stocks.

Cash-Based Investments

There isn't much that you can do to monitor the value of your cash-based investments, other than checking the balance of your savings account online and figuring out what a GIC or term deposit will be worth upon maturity.

Most major financial institutions in Canada offer Internet banking services that will allow you to check the balance of your savings account online.

When it comes to GICs and term deposits, keep in mind that these are investments that are taken out for a fixed period of time, anywhere from 30 days to five years or more. In most cases, you are earning a fixed rate of interest on the investment, and when the time period for the investment is up, it is said to mature. Hence, the key piece of information you want to know is its maturity value, or how much money you will get from the investment at the end of its term.

Usually you are given this information when you take out a GIC or term deposit at a financial institution. However, if you don't have that information readily available and would still like to know the value upon maturity, there are a few calculators on the Internet that will let you figure it out.

A useful starting point is the Web site belonging to Munica, a company that develops software for use by companies with Web sites. On their site they feature two GIC calculators. You can find them under the Products section, Web Financial Calculator Set.

The first one lets you do a basic calculation to find out how much you will get for a particular GIC investment upon maturity. In our example below we wanted to know the maturity value of investing $10,000 in a GIC for two years at the rate of 4%:

CHAPTER 9: Monitoring Your Performance

Fixed Rate GIC Calculator

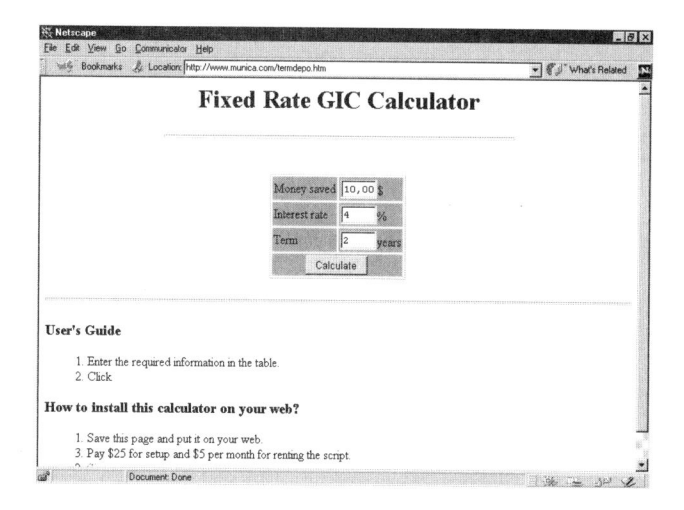

Money saved: 10,00 $
Interest rate: 4 %
Term: 2 years
[Calculate]

User's Guide

1. Enter the required information in the table.
2. Click

How to install this calculator on your web?

1. Save this page and put it on your web.
3. Pay $25 for setup and $5 per month for renting the script.

Munica's calculator instantly provided the details:

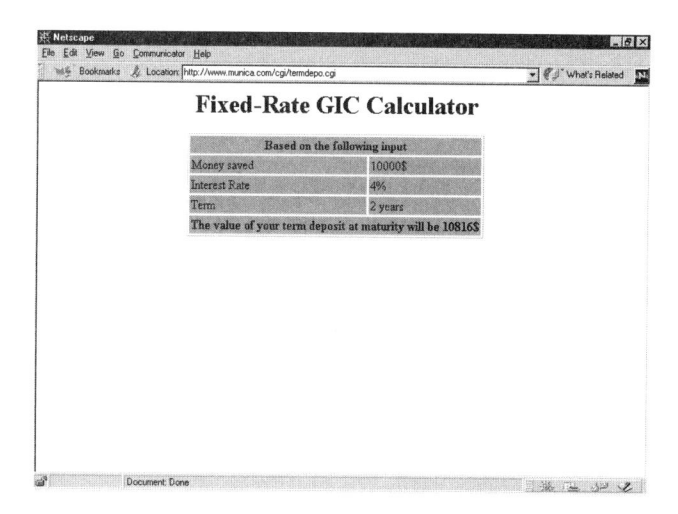

Fixed-Rate GIC Calculator

Based on the following input	
Money saved	10000$
Interest Rate	4%
Term	2 years
The value of your term deposit at maturity will be 10816$	

The second calculator lets you figure out how much your GIC/term deposit will be worth if there is a different rate of interest each year (as there are with many such products in the marketplace today):

Variable Rate GIC Calculator

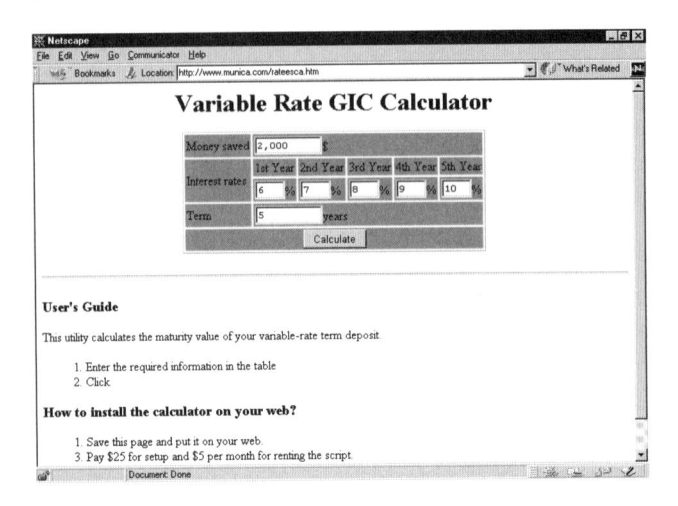

[Screenshot: Variable Rate GIC Calculator showing Money saved: 2,000$; Interest rates 1st Year 6%, 2nd Year 7%, 3rd Year 8%, 4th Year 9%, 5th Year 10%; Term: 5 years.

User's Guide

This utility calculates the maturity value of your variable-rate term deposit.

1. Enter the required information in the table
2. Click.

How to install the calculator on your web?

1. Save this page and put it on your web.
3. Pay $25 for setup and $5 per month for renting the script.]

If you're looking for a calculator that does this calculation for GIC/term deposit investments of less than a year, turn to Hepcoe Credit Union, which lets you do the same thing for GICs/term deposits of 30, 60, 90, 120, 180, or 270 days, in addition to various annual calculations:

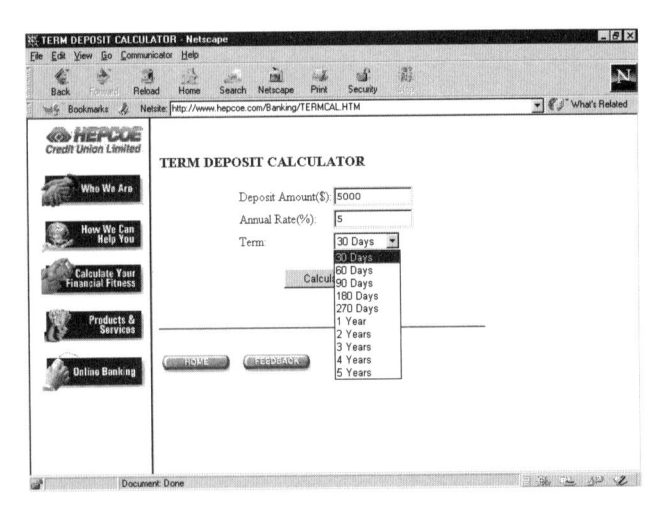

[Screenshot: Hepcoe Credit Union TERM DEPOSIT CALCULATOR with Deposit Amount($): 5000, Annual Rate(%): 5, Term dropdown showing 30 Days, 60 Days, 90 Days, 180 Days, 270 Days, 1 Year, 2 Years, 3 Years, 4 Years, 5 Years.]

Finally, Altamira's Web site has an online calculator called the "Capital Builder Calculator." You will find it under the Tool Kit section of their Resource Centre. You can use this calculator for a variety of purposes, such as to figure out how much an investment will be worth in the future.

When using this calculator, if you simply ignore the tax rate box and leave the payment box blank, you can use it for the same purpose as the calculators we described above:

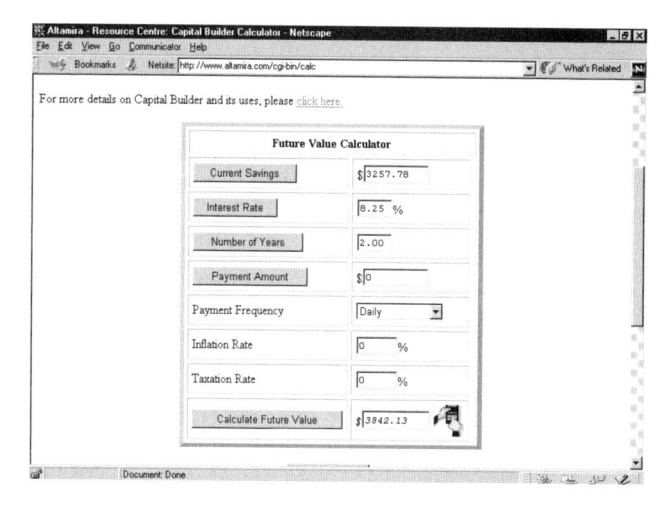

CHAPTER 9: Monitoring Your Performance

[Screenshot: Altamira Future Value Calculator showing Current Savings $3257.78, Interest Rate 6.25%, Number of Years 2.00, Payment Amount $0, Payment Frequency Daily, Inflation Rate 0%, Taxation Rate 0%, Calculate Future Value $3842.13]

In addition to using these online calculators, you should be aware that some financial organizations, such as Canada Trust, will let you examine the maturity value of your GIC or term deposit as part of their online banking services, particularly when the investment is included in your RRSP.

If you hold Canada Savings Bonds, you can figure out their value at maturity by visiting the federal government's Canada Savings Bond Web site. Simply indicate the particular CSB that you own and a valuation date, that is, today's date if you would like to know what it is worth now:

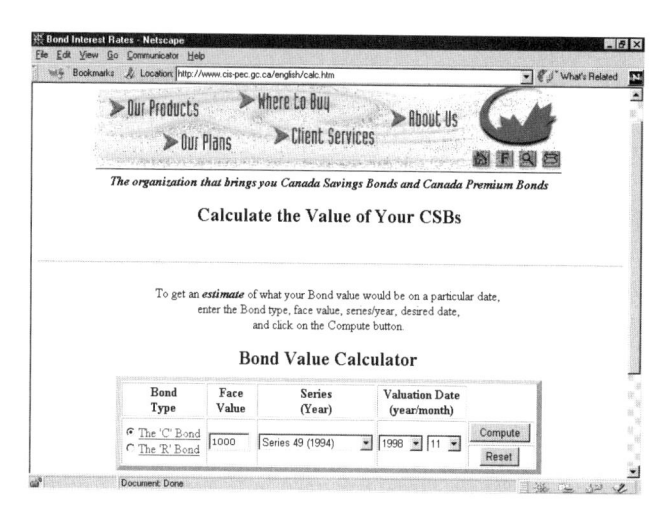

[Screenshot: Bond Value Calculator page showing Calculate the Value of Your CSBs, with fields for Bond Type ('C' Bond selected), Face Value 1000, Series 49 (1994), Valuation Date 1998/11]

Within a few seconds you will see the value of your bonds:

137

1999 MUTUAL FUNDS AND RRSPs ONLINE

Calculate the Value of Your CSBs

Bond Values: Calculation Results

You can print this page with the bond record table using your browser's print function.

Item	CSB Type	Face Value	Series (Year)	Selected Valuation Date	Estimated Value
1	The "C" Bond	1000	Series 49 (1994)	1998 - 11	1264.21
				Estimated Total	**1264.21**

1. The estimated values for Series 51 and 52 are based on the minimum guaranteed interest rates.
2. Actual values will vary according to the denominations of bonds held.
3. Bondholders redeeming Regular Interest Bonds in September and October will receive par value less two months' or one month's interest, respectively, and will receive a full year's interest on November 1.

Select another bond type, face value, series/year, desired date, and click again on the Compute button.

CSB Value Calculator

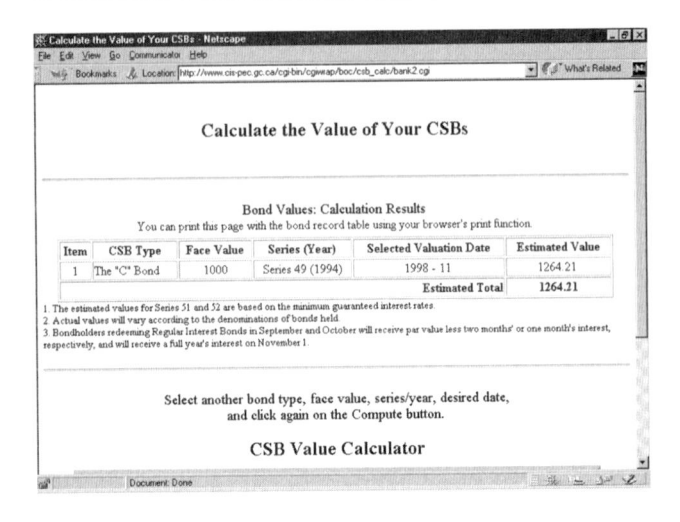

What's the bottom line? There is no shortage of useful calculators on the Web that will help you figure out how much you will earn on your cash-based investments.

Mutual Funds

What about your mutual funds? Is there anything you can do online to monitor how they are performing?

Of course there is! You can:

- look up the daily net asset values of any particular mutual fund in order to determine how the value compares to the previous day

- obtain simple reports and graphs to see how you are doing with a particular fund or to see how your fund has performed historically

- sign up with sophisticated "portfolio trackers" that let you see the overall value of your mutual fund holdings on a day-to-day basis, as well as analyze their performance through tables and graphs

- use individual "portfolio manager" software programs that allow you to do even more sophisticated tracking and analysis of your mutual fund holdings.

Over the next several pages we will provide examples of each of these applications.

CHAPTER 9 : Monitoring Your Performance

Daily Net Asset Values

Most Canadian mutual fund Web sites include a section where daily net asset values (NAVs) are posted, usually within a few hours of the close of the previous business day (see appendix C for more on NAVs). Consider, for example, this report from the AGF Group of Funds:

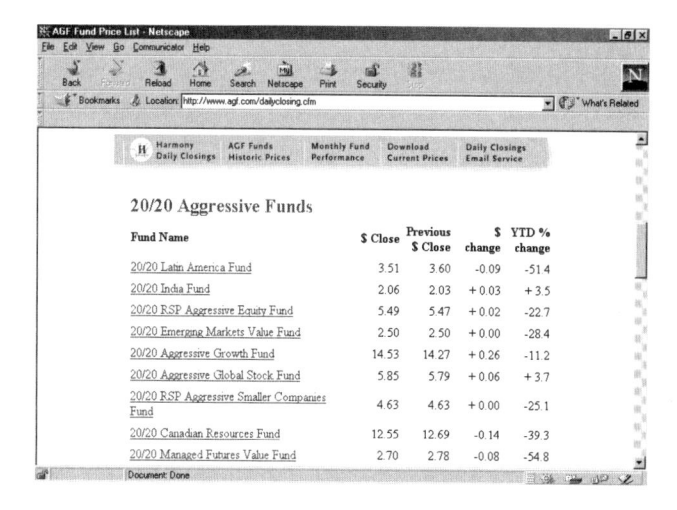

Fund Name	$ Close	Previous $ Close	$ change	YTD % change
20/20 Latin America Fund	3.51	3.60	-0.09	-51.4
20/20 India Fund	2.06	2.03	+0.03	+3.5
20/20 RSP Aggressive Equity Fund	5.49	5.47	+0.02	-22.7
20/20 Emerging Markets Value Fund	2.50	2.50	+0.00	-28.4
20/20 Aggressive Growth Fund	14.53	14.27	+0.26	-11.2
20/20 Aggressive Global Stock Fund	5.85	5.79	+0.06	+3.7
20/20 RSP Aggressive Smaller Companies Fund	4.63	4.63	+0.00	-25.1
20/20 Canadian Resources Fund	12.55	12.69	-0.14	-39.3
20/20 Managed Futures Value Fund	2.70	2.78	-0.08	-54.8

You can also get comprehensive listings of daily fund NAVs at such sites as The Fund Library, GLOBEfund, i|money, Quicken.ca, and CANOE. Each site lets you examine daily NAVs in a variety of ways.

You can use these sites to see how your fund is performing by comparing the daily NAV to the NAV on the date you purchased each mutual fund.

However, the use of such information can be deceiving. In many cases, income earned on various types of mutual funds is often added back into the fund, with a resultant increase in the number of units that you own.

Why is this so? When you purchase certain types of funds, you are asked if you want any income on the fund to be reinvested or if you would like it to be paid out to you. If reinvested, it is used to "purchase" a few more units for you. This additional "purchase" complicates the calculation so much that these simple calculators do not give a completely accurate picture of an investment. Many investors use the NAV as but one indicator of the overall performance of a fund.

1999 MUTUAL FUNDS AND RRSPs ONLINE

Simple Performance Reports and Graphs

Several Canadian mutual fund Web sites include tools that let you calculate or graphically view how your funds have performed over time.

At the Phillips, Hager & North Web site, for example, you can find out how much an investment in their funds will have grown over time; they call this their "what-if" analysis.

On the following screen we've asked to see how an investment in their Money Market fund would have increased in value from January 1993 to September 1998:

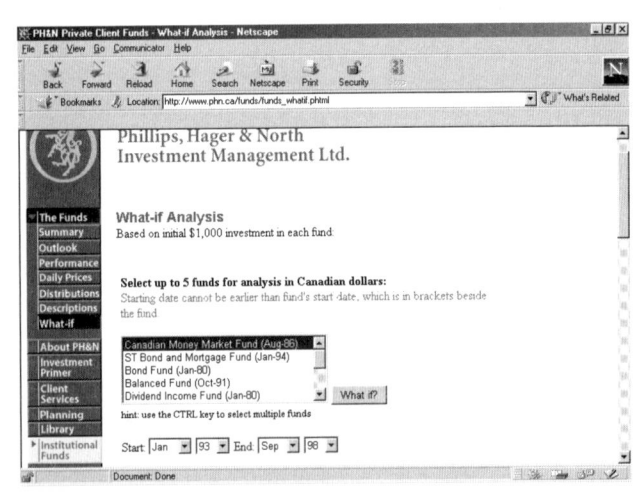

We were advised that every $1,000 invested in this fund at the start of 1993 would have grown in value to $1,290.31, for an effective annual rate of return of 4.6%.

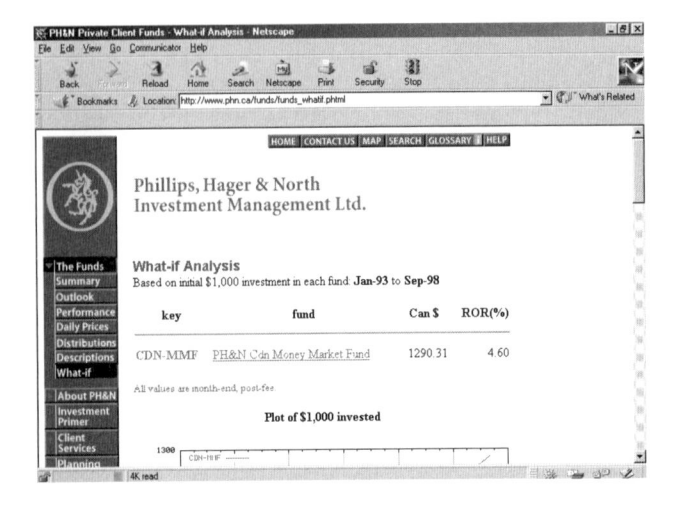

CHAPTER 9 : Monitoring Your Performance

The Royal Bank Web site lets you do the same thing, but also allows you to view the results in a simple graph that charts the performance of a particular fund. You provide details on the date that you invested in the fund as well as the amount that you invested.

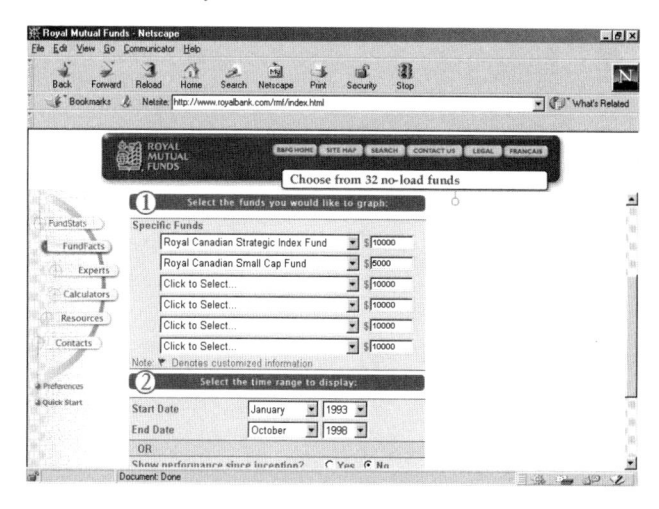

Within a few seconds, you are provided with a graph that shows you the fluctuations in the value of your fund investment over time as well as the estimated value of the investment and the average annual rate of return on the fund during that time period:

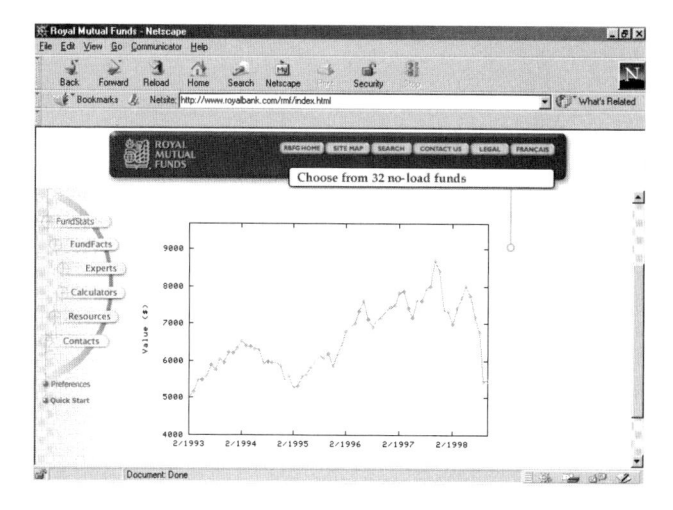

1999 MUTUAL FUNDS AND RRSPs ONLINE

Finally, AGF lets you prepare similar graphs for up to three investments at once:

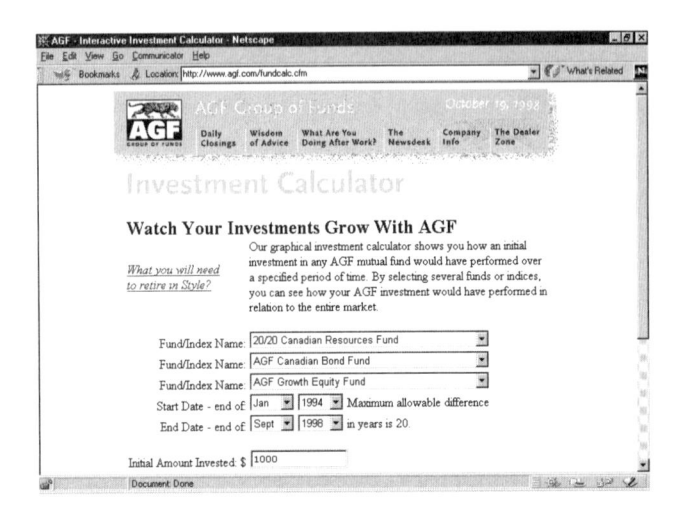

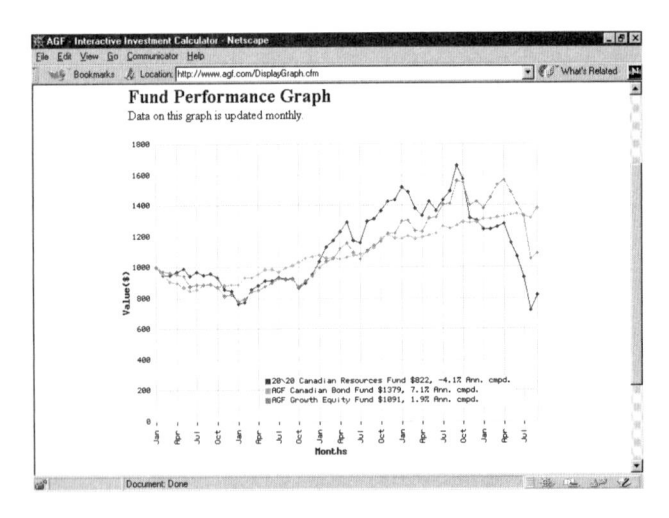

These are but a few examples of the tools provided directly by the organizations that offer mutual funds. Be sure to check the company Web sites of the funds you own, since they also might offer tools to help you to assess your portfolio's performance.

However, there are a few downsides to these simple performance reports and graphs:

- Your analysis cannot take into account multiple investments in the same fund over a period of time. The calculations and graphs described above simply recognize the change in the value of your investment over a period of time. If you invested in the fund again in the subsequent year and again the following year, the graphing that you do will not show that fact; you must run a separate graph for each investment you made.

- The Web sites described above only let you do an analysis with the funds they sell. For obvious competitive reasons, the Royal Bank doesn't let you chart or view performance for AGF funds and vice versa.

- These tools do not allow you to save your graph under your own name or some other identifying factor, meaning that you must enter your investment data each time you visit.

Even with these limitations, however, these simple tools are an effective and straightforward means of graphically viewing the performance of your mutual fund investments.

Portfolio Trackers

A more sophisticated way to monitor the performance of your mutual fund investments involves the use of "portfolio trackers."

A number of independent financial sites—The Fund Library and GLOBEfund in particular—provide the capability to track the overall performance and value of all of your mutual fund holdings on a day-to-day basis.

You can, for example, set up an account at The Fund Library to use their Personal Fund Monitor. After you create a "library card" to obtain a user-ID and password, you simply add the funds that you own to your personal list. You can then go back to The Fund Library at any time and view various key indicators of your mutual fund holdings, such as rankings for less than one year and opinions given about the funds by various people including Gordon Pape and Duff Young.

1999 MUTUAL FUNDS AND RRSPs ONLINE

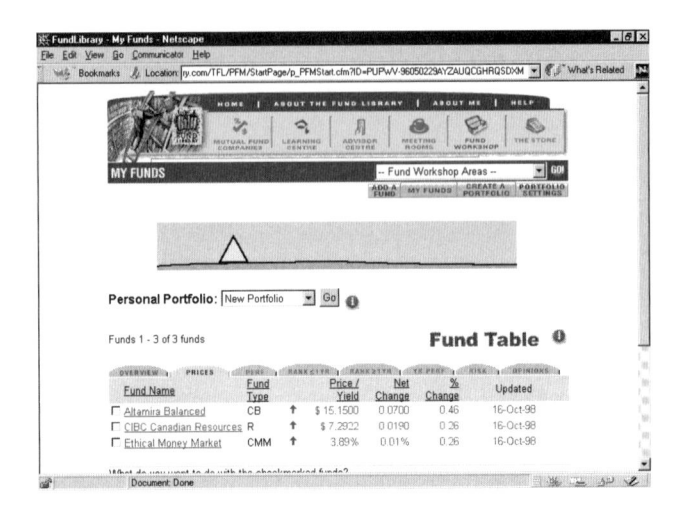

You can increase your understanding of the performance of your funds by taking advantage of the "Portfolio Tracker" at the same Web site. The Portfolio Tracker allows you to track your actual fund purchases, monitor their daily performance, and view various reports (such as the gain/loss report) specific to your portfolio.

To set yourself up on the Portfolio Tracker, you fill out a form to obtain a library card to get a user-ID and password. After doing that, you need to set up your portfolio. You do this by first selecting the fund company that manages the fund:

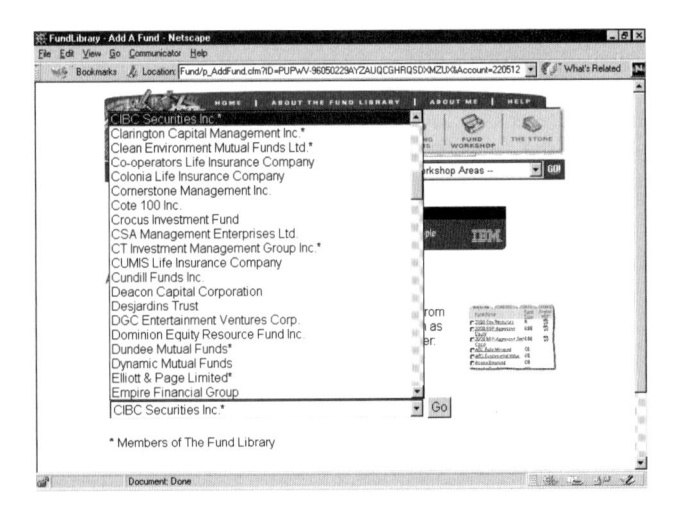

CHAPTER 9 : Monitoring Your Performance

You then select the mutual fund that you purchased from that company:

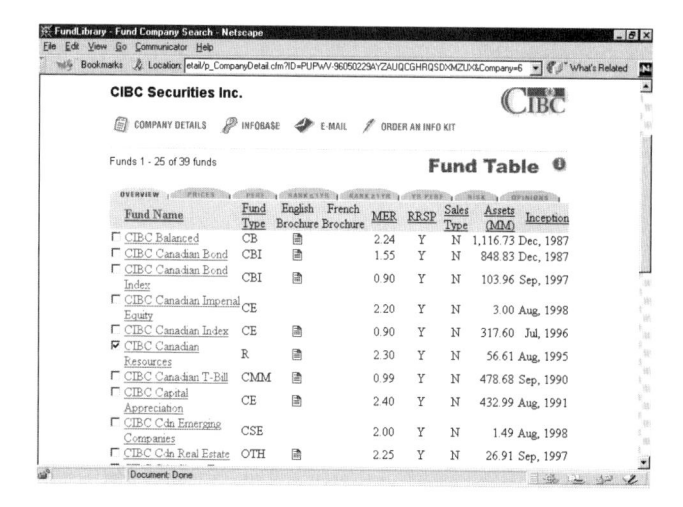

CIBC Securities Inc.

COMPANY DETAILS   INFOBASE   E-MAIL   ORDER AN INFO KIT

Funds 1 - 25 of 39 funds

Fund Table

Fund Name	Fund Type	English Brochure	French Brochure	MER	RRSP	Sales Type	Assets (MM)	Inception
CIBC Balanced	CB			2.24	Y	N	1,116.73	Dec, 1987
CIBC Canadian Bond	CBI			1.55	Y	N	848.83	Dec, 1987
CIBC Canadian Bond Index	CBI			0.90	Y	N	103.96	Sep, 1997
CIBC Canadian Imperial Equity	CE			2.20	Y	N	3.00	Aug, 1998
CIBC Canadian Index	CE			0.90	Y	N	317.60	Jul, 1996
CIBC Canadian Resources	R			2.30	Y	N	56.61	Aug, 1995
CIBC Canadian T-Bill	CMM			0.99	Y	N	478.68	Sep, 1990
CIBC Capital Appreciation	CE			2.40	Y	N	432.99	Aug, 1991
CIBC Cdn Emerging Companies	CSE			2.00	Y	N	1.49	Aug, 1998
CIBC Cdn Real Estate	OTH			2.25	Y	N	26.91	Sep, 1997

Next, you provide more details about your fund, such as the date of purchase, the number of mutual fund units that you purchased, and the cost per unit. If you do not know the cost per unit, you can use the Lookup Price feature to find it. If you made multiple purchases over time in the fund, you have to enter each of these transactions separately.

This precise information is necessary, because The Fund Library will use it to provide the exact value of your mutual fund holdings at any time. You will also have the ability to track the performance of your funds from the date you purchased them to the current point in time. The information you provide for each fund transaction is summarized in the Transaction History Report:

1999 MUTUAL FUNDS AND RRSPs ONLINE

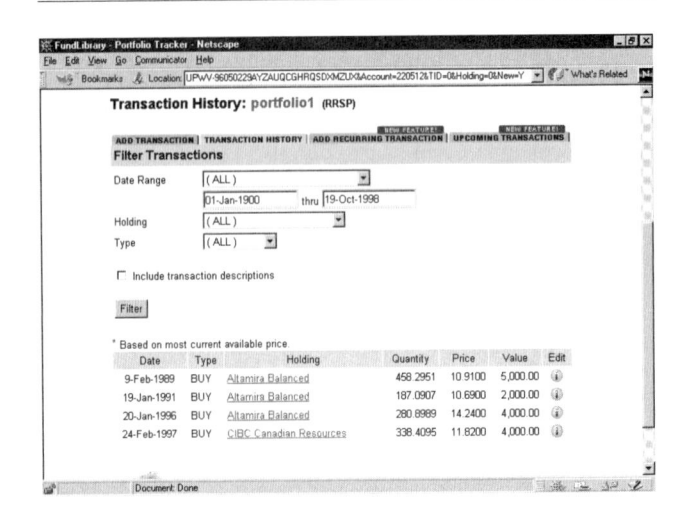

Once you do this for all your mutual fund purchases, you can view various reports that track your portfolio. Two such reports are the Portfolio Report, which gives the current value of your mutual funds:

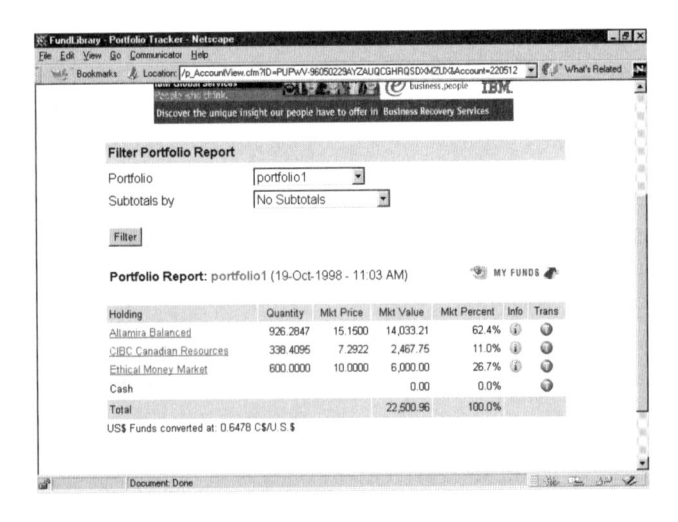

and the Gain/Loss report:

CHAPTER 9 : Monitoring Your Performance

Filter Gain/Loss Report

Portfolio: portfolio1

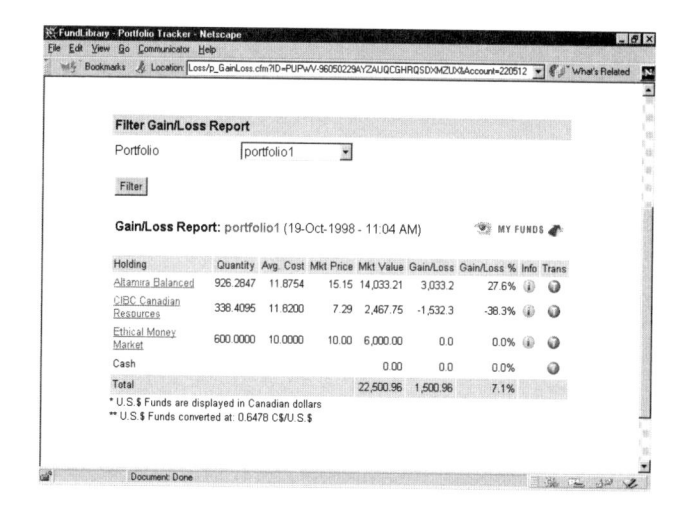

[Filter]

Gain/Loss Report: portfolio1 (19-Oct-1998 - 11:04 AM)   MY FUNDS

Holding	Quantity	Avg. Cost	Mkt Price	Mkt Value	Gain/Loss	Gain/Loss %	Info	Trans
Altamira Balanced	926.2847	11.8754	15.15	14,033.21	3,033.2	27.6%		
CIBC Canadian Resources	338.4095	11.8200	7.29	2,467.75	-1,532.3	-38.3%		
Ethical Money Market	600.0000	10.0000	10.00	6,000.00	0.0	0.0%		
Cash				0.00	0.0	0.0%		
Total				22,500.96	1,500.96	7.1%		

* U.S.$ Funds are displayed in Canadian dollars
** U.S.$ Funds converted at: 0.6478 C$/U.S.$

The *Globe and Mail*'s GLOBEfund site also provides the ability to prepare some very useful reports on your fund holdings using your "Fundlist."

Once you have set up the listing of funds that you wish to track, creating what is then referred to as your Fundlist, you can quickly obtain a report on the value and performance of your funds. One of the key benefits of GLOBEfund is that you can sort the report in different ways. For example, you can choose to see which funds are performing best in the short term, over one, three, or five years, or by the most recent percentage change in fund values:

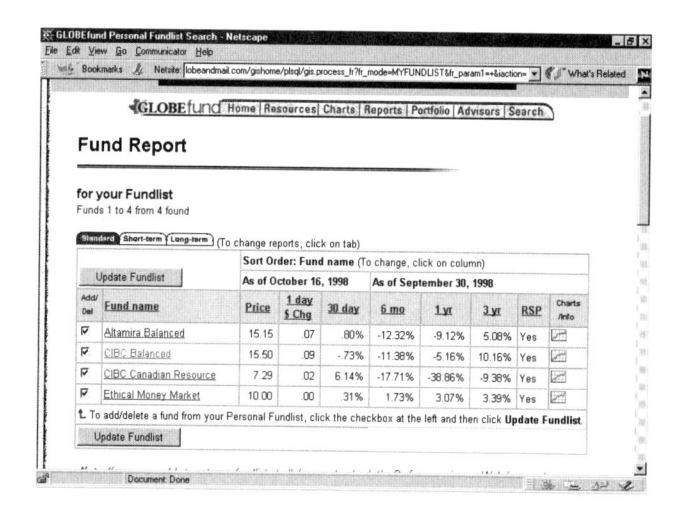

GLOBEfund Home | Resources | Charts | Reports | Portfolio | Advisors | Search

Fund Report

for your Fundlist
Funds 1 to 4 from 4 found

Standard *Short-term* *Long-term* (To change reports, click on tab)

[Update Fundlist]

Sort Order: **Fund name** (To change, click on column)
As of October 16, 1998   As of September 30, 1998

Add/Del	Fund name	Price	1 day $ Chg	30 day	6 mo	1 yr	3 yr	RSP	Charts /Info
☑	Altamira Balanced	15.15	.07	.80%	-12.32%	-9.12%	5.08%	Yes	
☑	CIBC Balanced	15.50	.09	-.73%	-11.38%	-5.16%	10.16%	Yes	
☑	CIBC Canadian Resource	7.29	.02	6.14%	-17.71%	-38.86%	-9.38%	Yes	
☑	Ethical Money Market	10.00	.00	.31%	1.73%	3.07%	3.39%	Yes	

⇡ To add/delete a fund from your Personal Fundlist, click the checkbox at the left and then click **Update Fundlist**.

[Update Fundlist]

1999 MUTUAL FUNDS AND RRSPs ONLINE

In addition, you can chart the performance of any particular fund against other funds that you own and compare it against other factors such as the overall performance of funds on the TSE:

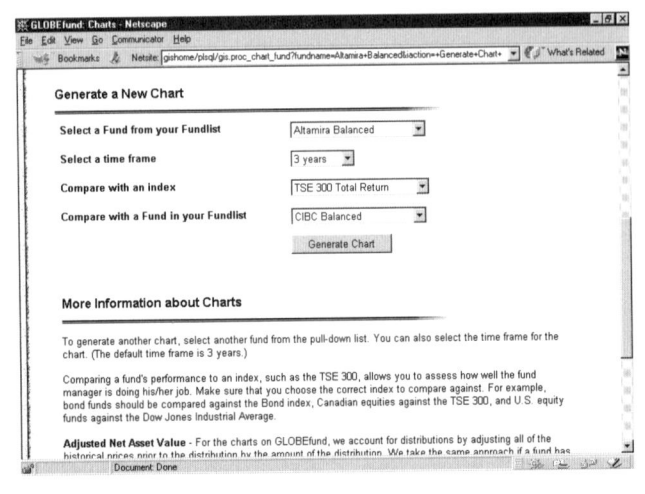

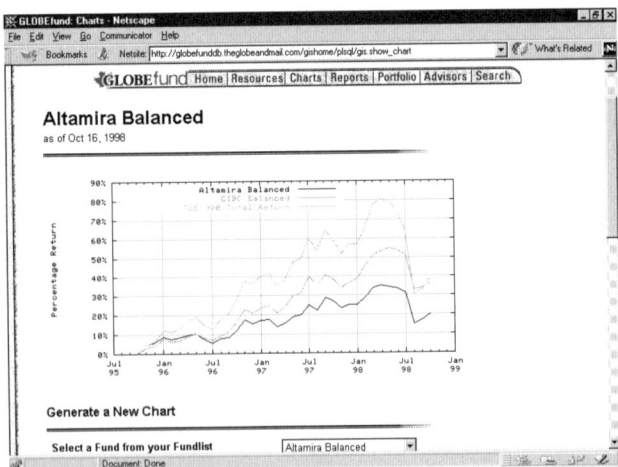

The GLOBEfund site also has a portfolio tracker, which allows you to track your actual mutual fund holdings, transaction by transaction. Similar portfolio tracking capabilities can be found at the Web sites of i|money and Quicken.ca.

Finally, check out some of the Southam newspaper Web sites such as *The Vancouver Sun*. Many include a portfolio manager that you can use to track your mutual funds. You can get a full list of Southam newspapers at the Southam Web site.

Portfolio Management Software

The last method of monitoring mutual fund performance on the Web is to use portfolio management software, which runs as a separate program, not in your Web browser.

Such programs let you examine mutual fund data faster than through a Web browser, often feature extensive historical information, offer accounting capabilities that let you easily track each and every mutual fund sale and purchase, and generally offer a wealth of other features not offered by the tools we've looked at so far.

One of the best examples of this type of software is PALTrak from Portfolio Analytics. On their Web site they describe the product as "Canada's most comprehensive mutual fund sales, analysis and research software," and that claim is not a stretch.

You can download a fully functional version of the software from the Portfolio Analytics Web site. The program is fully usable, but contains outdated data. If you want the most recent data, you can purchase the most recent month's fund information for $59 or buy an annual subscription for $399.

1999 MUTUAL FUNDS AND RRSPs ONLINE

What can you do with this program? First and foremost, the program contains comprehensive information on all available Canadian mutual funds, including details on performance over time, most recent NAVs, and other useful information:

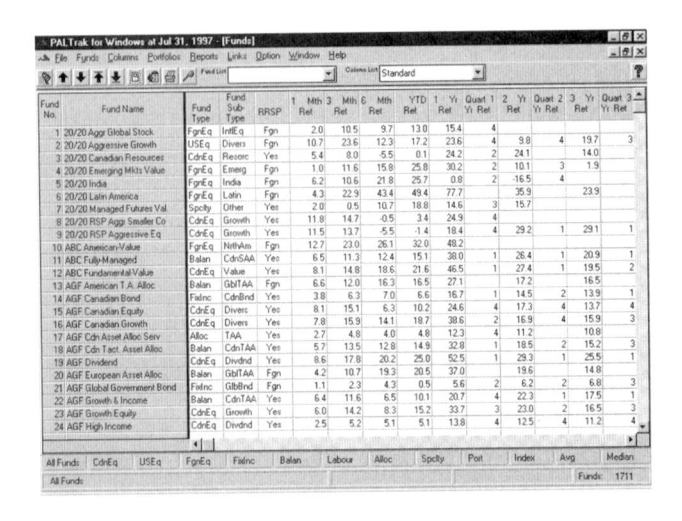

To create your own portfolio, you simply highlight the particular funds that you own:

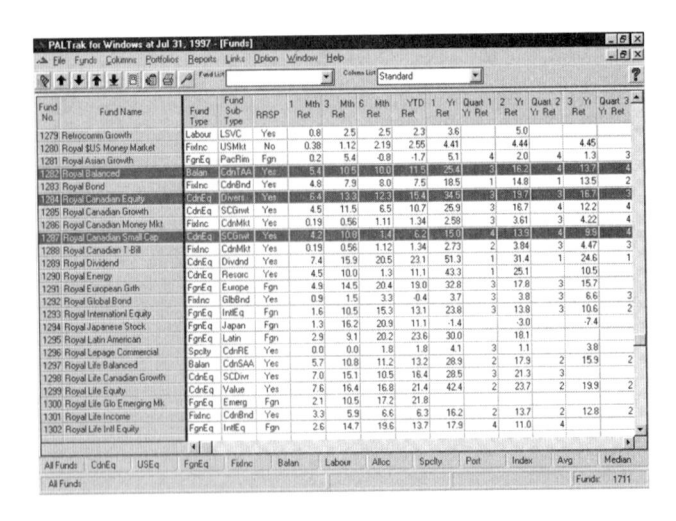

You then need to provide the transaction details for each fund that you own, much like you need to do at The Fund Library site:

CHAPTER 9 : Monitoring Your Performance

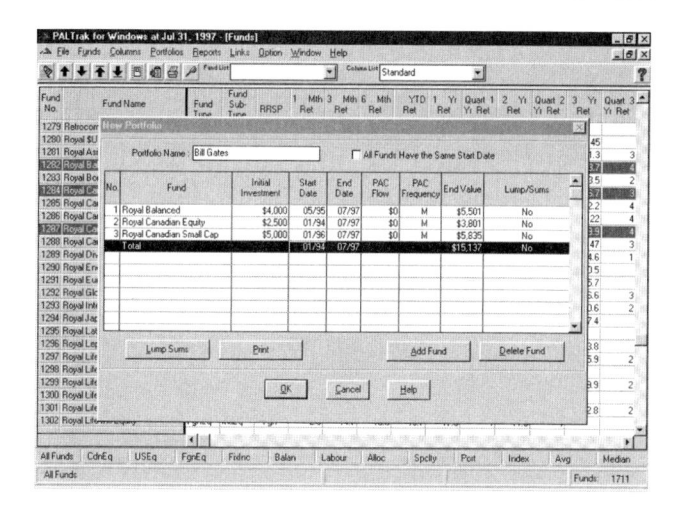

Once you have done this, you can use PALTrak to analyze your portfolio from a variety of perspectives. For example, on the following screen the performance of funds held by an investor is being compared to the returns that would have been earned had the money been invested in a Canada Savings Bond or five-year GIC:

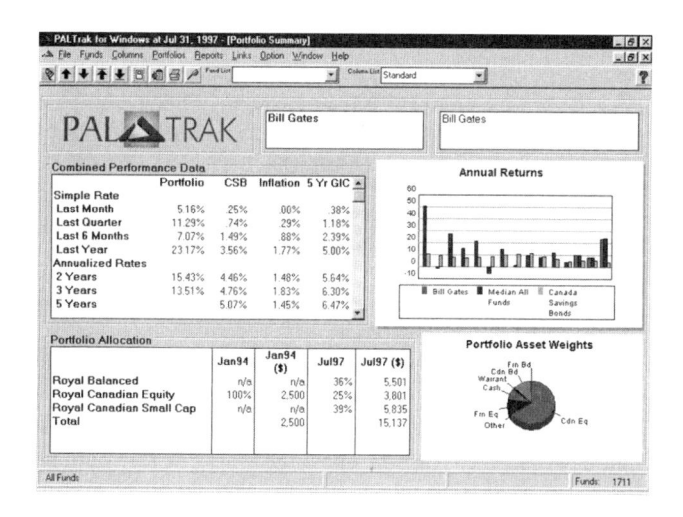

On the following screen we've asked for a breakdown of the fund investments by fund type. The results will tell you whether your fund investments match the investment objectives that you established earlier:

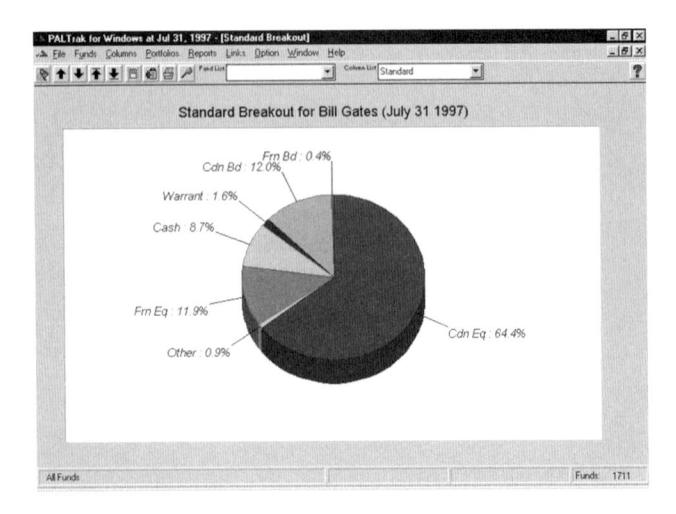

1999 MUTUAL FUNDS AND RRSPs ONLINE

[Screenshot: PALTrak for Windows - Standard Breakout for Bill Gates (July 31 1997) pie chart showing: Cdn Eq: 64.4%, Cdn Bd: 12.0%, Frn Eq: 11.9%, Cash: 8.7%, Warrant: 1.6%, Other: 0.9%, Frn Bd: 0.4%]

And below we've asked PALTrak to give us an overview of the types of holdings found in our equity mutual fund investments:

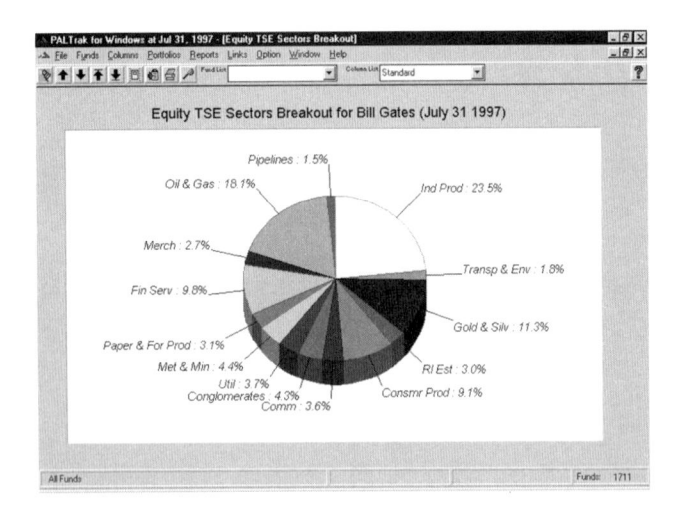

[Screenshot: PALTrak for Windows - Equity TSE Sectors Breakout for Bill Gates (July 31 1997) pie chart showing: Ind Prod: 23.5%, Oil & Gas: 18.1%, Gold & Silv: 11.3%, Fin Serv: 9.8%, Consmr Prod: 9.1%, Met & Min: 4.4%, Conglomerates: 4.3%, Util: 3.7%, Comm: 3.6%, Paper & For Prod: 3.1%, Rl Est: 3.0%, Merch: 2.7%, Transp & Env: 1.9%, Pipelines: 1.5%]

Through the use of increasingly sophisticated programs such as PALTrak, you will not only have a better understanding of how your funds are doing, you will also find out if they match the investment objectives that you had previously set for yourself.

Stocks

In addition to cash-based investments and mutual funds, you may have placed some of your money in stocks. There are a number of possibilities for tracking the performance of your shares on the Internet.

Online Stock Quotes

There is no shortage of Web sites that you can use to obtain recent stock quotes. Most of the services that we describe in this section offer "15- or 20-minute delayed" quotes for free. This means that the most current stock price that you can see is from 15 or 20 minutes ago.

Free real-time quotes are available from a number of sites, most of which require you to register. One of the most popular services on the Web for obtaining real-time stock quotes is Quote.com. For most investors who simply want to track how their stocks are doing, 20-minute delayed quotes are more than sufficient. More serious investors who need up-to-the-second stock prices may want to consider the real-time information services provided by sites such as Quote.com. As you can see in the table below, there are many sites that offer delayed stock quotes; many of these also include free real-time quotes such as QuotesCanada.com. Most of the Web sites offer quotes from both Canadian and American exchanges.

Examples of Web Sites That Provide Free Stock Quotes

Canada Stockwatch	chart.canada-stockwatch.com
Canada Trust	www.canadatrust.com
CANOE	www.canoe.ca/Investment
Canadian Stock Market Reporter Inc.	www.canstock.com
Carlson On-line Services	www.carlsononline.com
Charles Schwab	www.schwab.com
CheckFree Quote Server	www.secapl.com/cgi-bin/qs
E*Trade	www.etrade.com
E*Trade Canada	www.canada.etrade.com
freerealtime.com	www.freerealtime.com

1999 MUTUAL FUNDS AND RRSPs ONLINE

InfoSpace.com	www.infospace.com
Market Guide	www.marketguide.com
Money.com	www.money.com
Quote.com	www.quote.com
QuotesCanada.com	www.quotescanada.com
Standard and Poor's	www.personalwealth.com
Stockpoint	www.stockpoint.com
Telenium	www.telenium.ca
Thomson Real Time Quotes	www.thomsonrtq.com

CANOE (Canadian Online Explorer) is one of dozens of Web sites that provide free access to delayed stock prices:

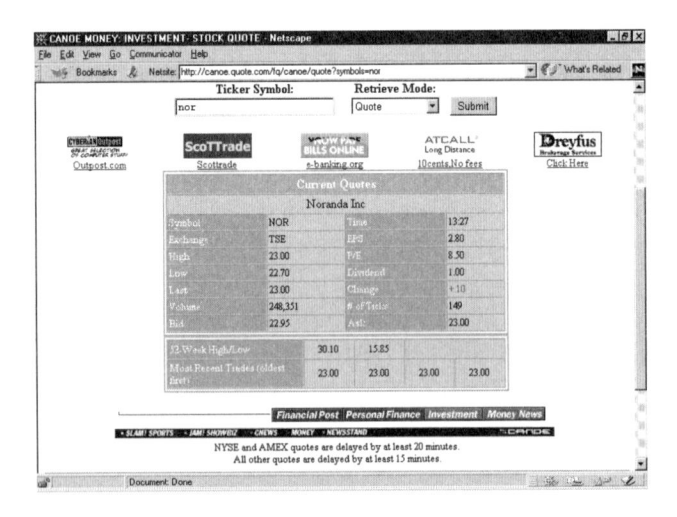

An increasing number of sites are setting up services that allow you to quickly obtain prices for stocks that you own, without having to manually type in the stock symbols each time you visit.

For example, CT Securities, a Canada Trust company, lets you set up a personal portfolio so that you can track the most recent quotes for up to twenty different stocks. Using the CT Market Partner Web site to set up your own portfolio is easy, and it's free:

CHAPTER 9 : Monitoring Your Performance

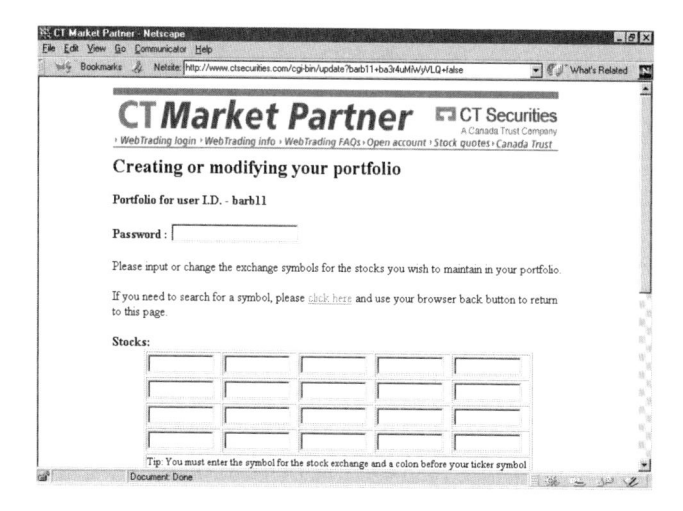

If you don't know the symbol of a stock you want to monitor, the site provides a simple way to look it up:

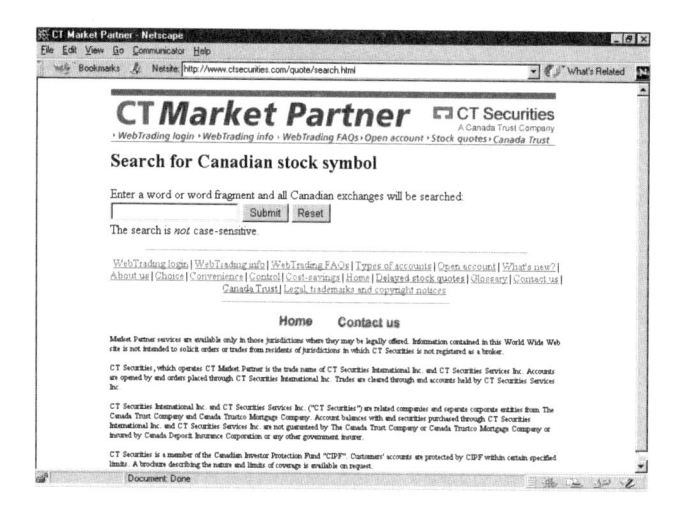

Once you have established your portfolio, you can return at any time to obtain the most recent (15-minute delayed) value of your shares:

155

1999 MUTUAL FUNDS AND RRSPs ONLINE

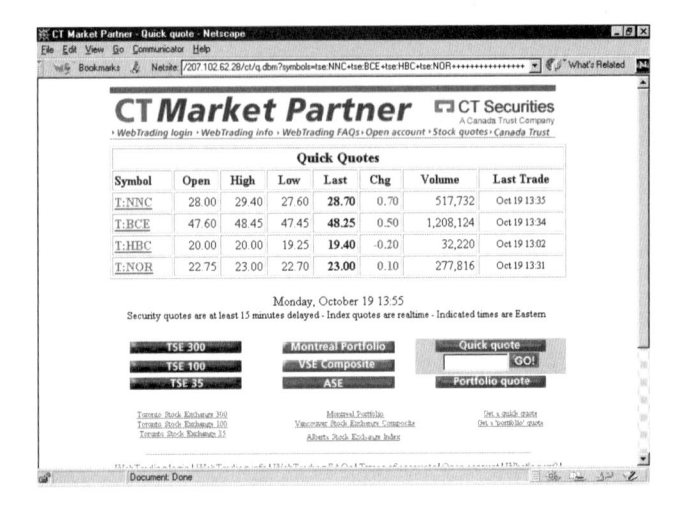

You can also obtain additional details for any stock in your portfolio, including a list of the most recent trades and the year's high and low prices on the stock:

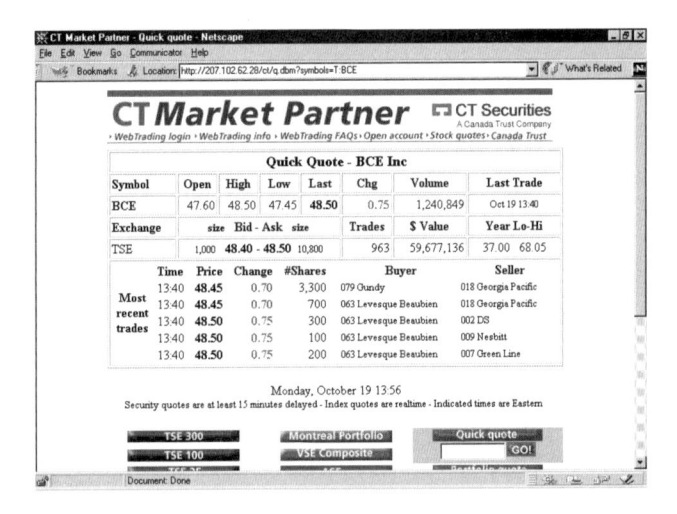

You can do the same thing at the CANOE site:

CHAPTER 9: Monitoring Your Performance

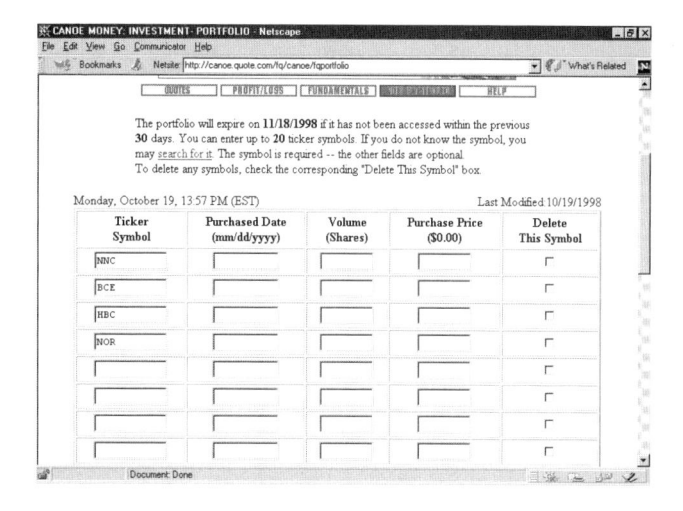

You can also return at any time to see the most recent trading prices:

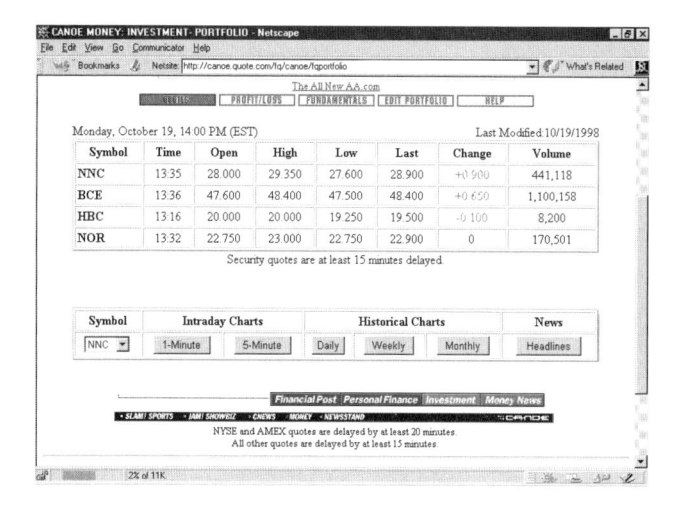

One of the most useful stock tracking services on the Internet is the Web site run by Carlson On-line Services. Carlson allows you to quickly find stock prices, news information, news releases, and other information for publicly traded Canadian companies.

Type in the stock symbol (a lookup capability is provided if you don't know it), and you are given a page that provides access to information on the Internet about the company. This site is extremely useful when you want to research a specific publicly traded Canadian company:

1999 MUTUAL FUNDS AND RRSPs ONLINE

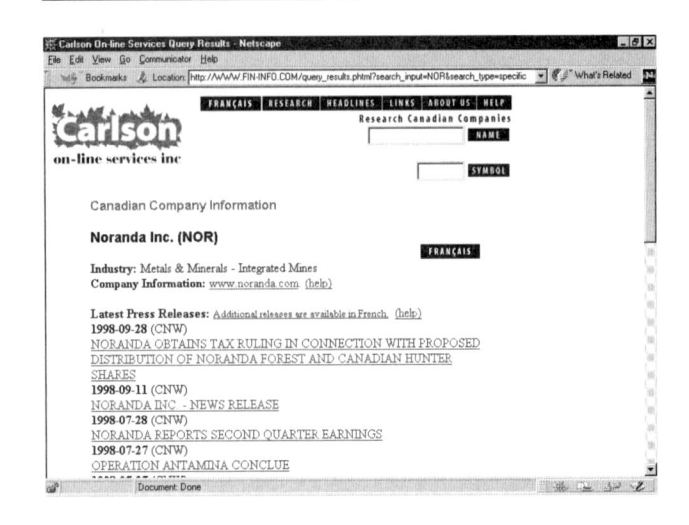

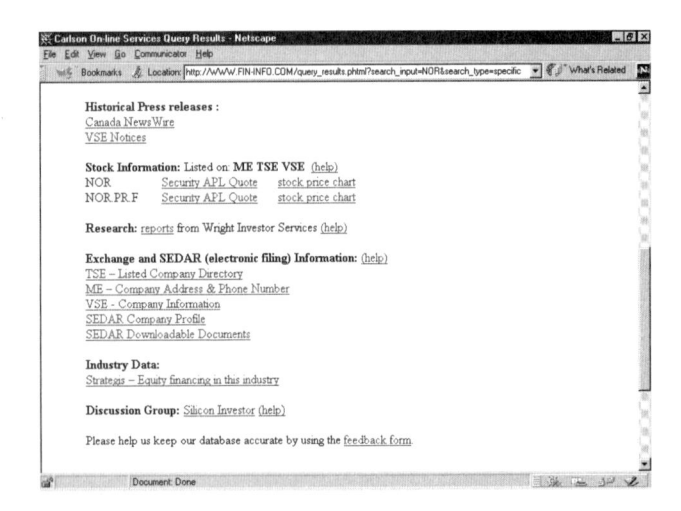

Online Stock Portfolio Managers

When we looked at mutual funds earlier in the chapter, we saw that there were a number of Web sites that let you set up detailed information about your portfolio, such as the number of units purchased of each fund. This lets you examine the total value of your mutual fund holdings at any time.

It should come as no surprise that a number of increasingly sophisticated "stock portfolio manager" programs are becoming available on investment Web sites throughout the Internet.

CHAPTER 9: Monitoring Your Performance

A Web site called Stockpoint, for example, lets you create a number of different portfolios. Simply enter the stocks you want to monitor, including the quantities you own and the commission you paid:

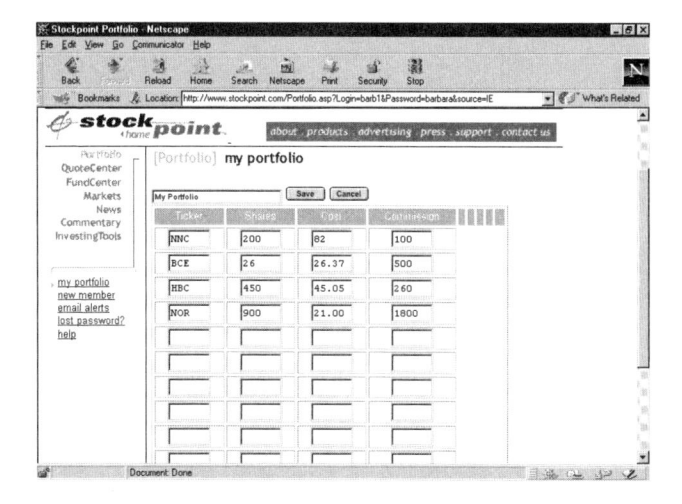

You can then examine, at any time, a report summarizing how well you are doing with these stocks:

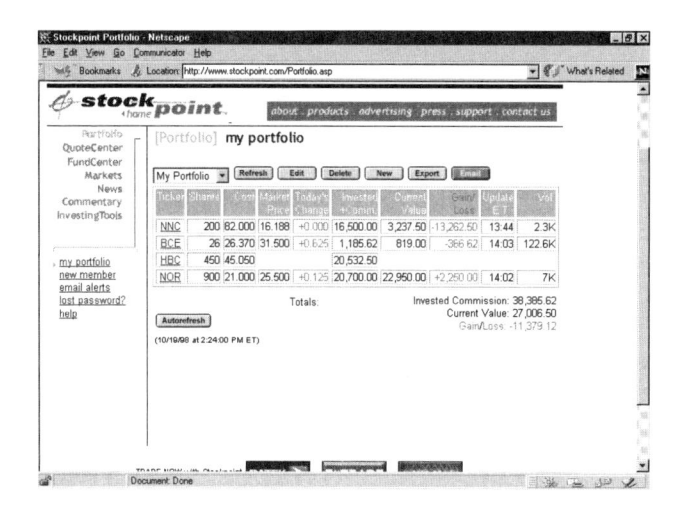

Similarly, E*Trade Canada offers a commercial portfolio manager service, seen on the next screen. If you sign up with E*Trade Canada in order to sell or purchase mutual funds or stocks, you can take advantage of their service:

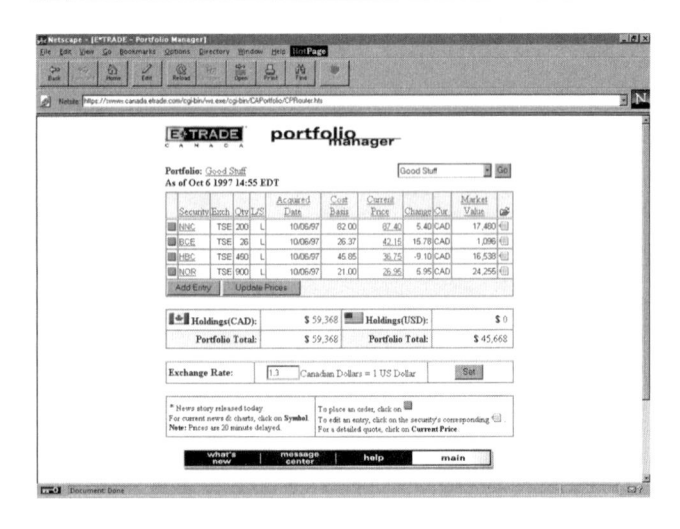

The features available on these online stock portfolio managers are constantly changing. For example, StockSmart lets you set up an "alert" so that you are notified by e-mail (or pager, if you prefer) if a certain stock price falls above or below a certain amount:

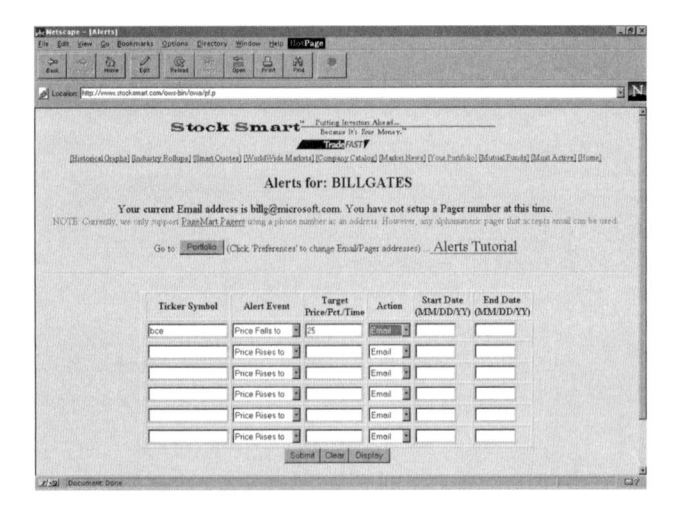

StockSmart will also allow you to "download" your portfolio information so that you can use the data in a spreadsheet or other program on your computer.

Integrated Software Programs

What if you want to use only one piece of software to track all of your investments?

Telenium, a Canadian software company, provides the Personal Portfolio program, which allows you to obtain an up-to-date valuation of your investment portfolio, including your stocks and mutual funds.

Simply key in the stocks and mutual funds that you own, and then press a button to get an up-to-date report. Current information is then retrieved through your Internet connection:

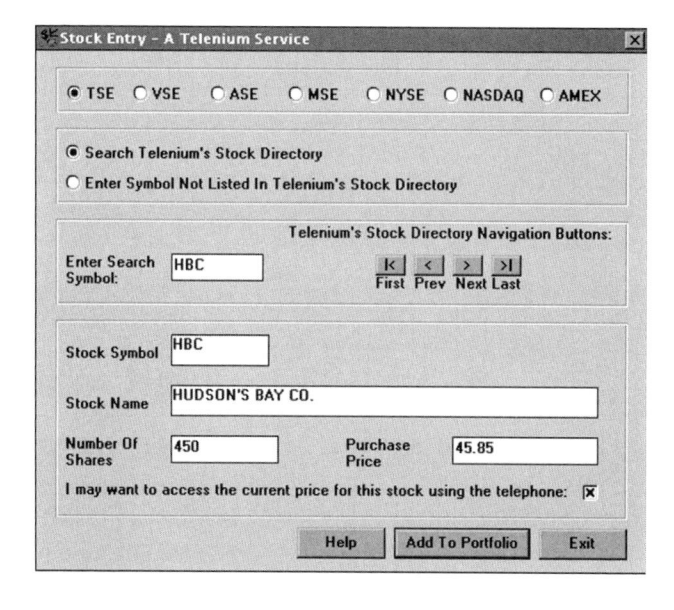

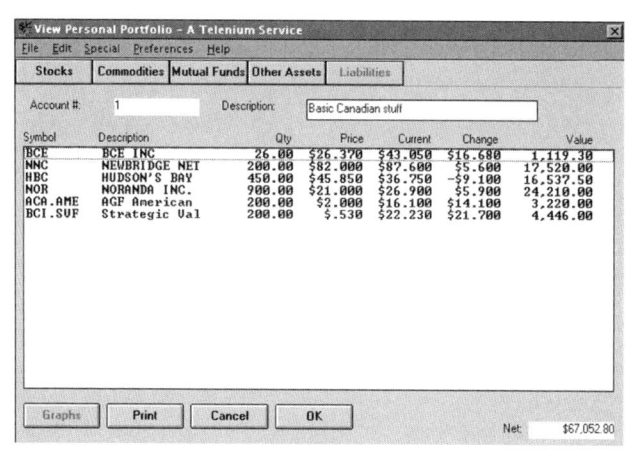

The Future of Investment Tracking Online

Finally, it's useful to look at a software program called Quicken for a glimpse of how sophisticated things have become.

Quicken is a computer program used for personal financial management or for business accounting. It is one of the most popular personal computer programs in the world.

Quicken also includes tools for investment management. Quicken 98 and 99 feature the ability to retrieve, through the Internet, up-to-date Canadian mutual fund, stock, and other investment values, thus making it an extremely useful investment portfolio manager.

The program provides users with many different options for managing their investments. For example, you can enter any number of investments into any number of portfolios:

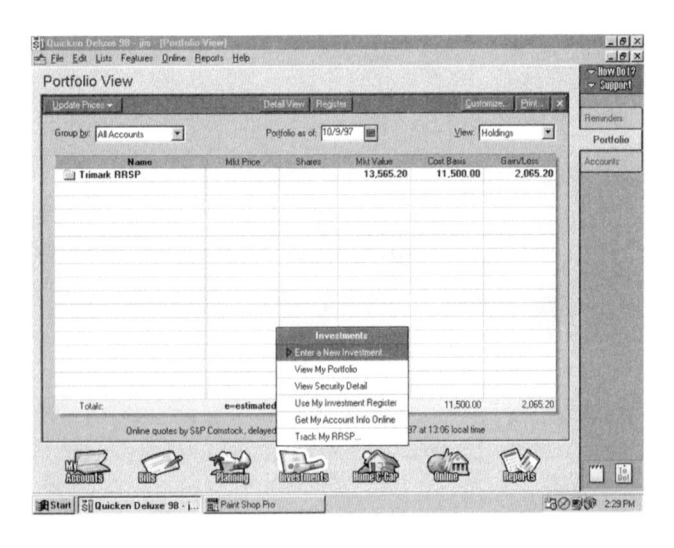

Each of your investments can be placed into categories that you define, thus helping you to keep things organized. For example, in our hypothetical case on page 163, we'll list our Royal Bank RRSPs in one "folder" and Trimark RRSPs in another:

CHAPTER 9 : Monitoring Your Performance

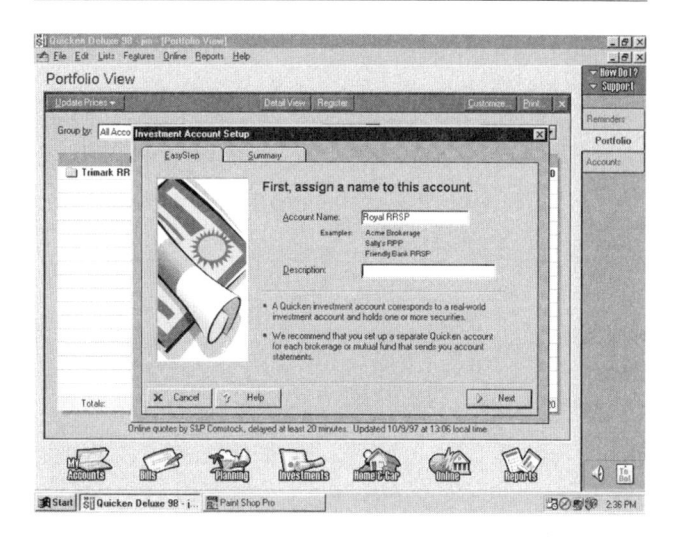

![Screenshot of Quicken Deluxe 98 Investment Account Setup dialog showing "First, assign a name to this account." with Account Name field filled in as "Royal RRSP"]

The program allows you to assign investments to an RRSP category. Alternatively, you can indicate that they are for general investment purposes only. This will help you to keep different investments separate for purposes of your income tax return:

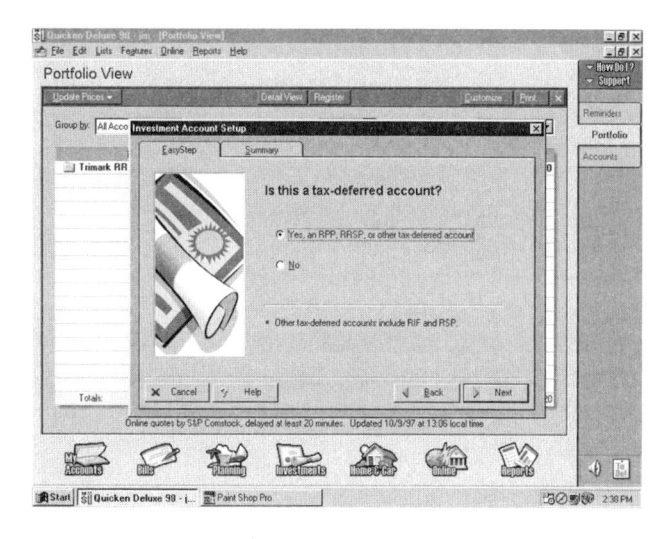

![Screenshot of Quicken Deluxe 98 Investment Account Setup dialog showing "Is this a tax-deferred account?" with "Yes, an RPP, RRSP, or other tax-deferred account" selected]

When you set up your investments on Quicken, you can input the "ticker symbol" for a stock, mutual fund, or other financial investment. These are symbols used throughout the investment industry. The program includes a lookup feature to help you if you do not know the symbol for a particular investment. These symbols are

1999 MUTUAL FUNDS AND RRSPs ONLINE

used to look up the market value of your investments through the Internet.

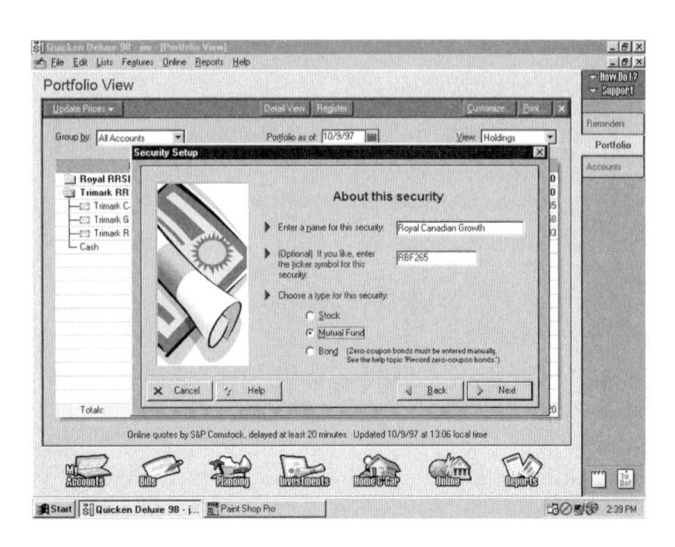

You can also use Quicken to keep track of how diversified your portfolio is. For example, you can identify whether a particular investment was for purposes of growth or income or whether you would classify it as a high-risk or low-risk investment. This can become very useful later when running the reports the program allows you to generate, for it can help you understand if your investment profile in terms of risk matches your risk objectives and whether your mix of growth and income investments matches the objectives that you set out earlier.

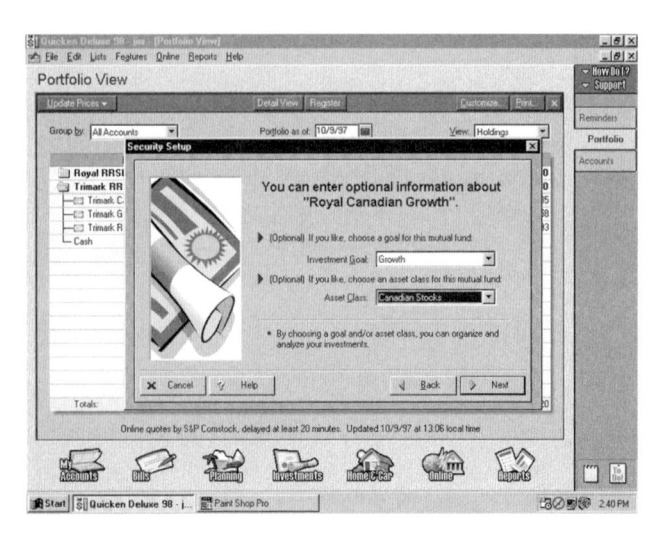

CHAPTER 9 : Monitoring Your Performance

Not only that, but the Quicken software is a full-fledged portfolio manager, in that it lets you build an exact record of your investment transactions. For each and every investment, you enter the date of purchase, the cost, and the commission paid. This allows you to view the performance of your investment later on:

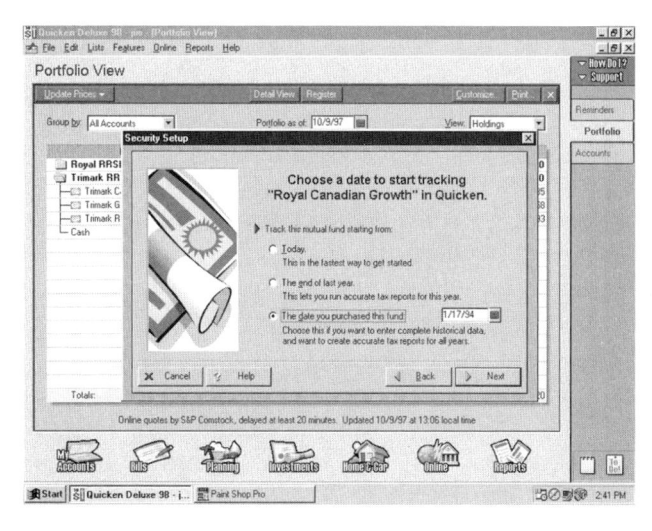

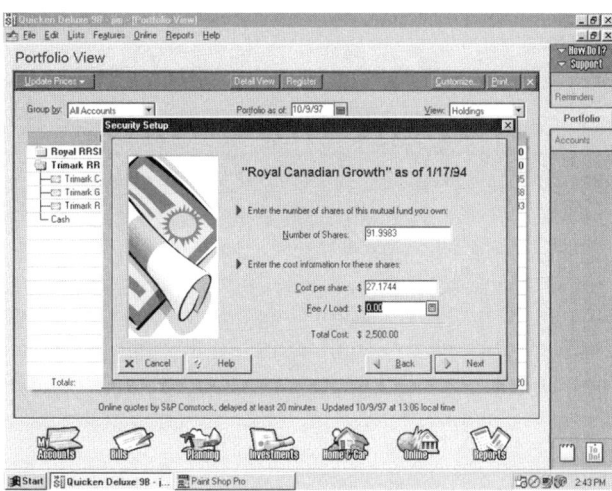

Once you have done this, you have a concise summary of your investments. Want updated market values? Simply press "Update," and the Quicken software will use your Internet connection to get them. This will generate a report that tells you how your investments are performing based on their current market value:

165

1999 MUTUAL FUNDS AND RRSPs ONLINE

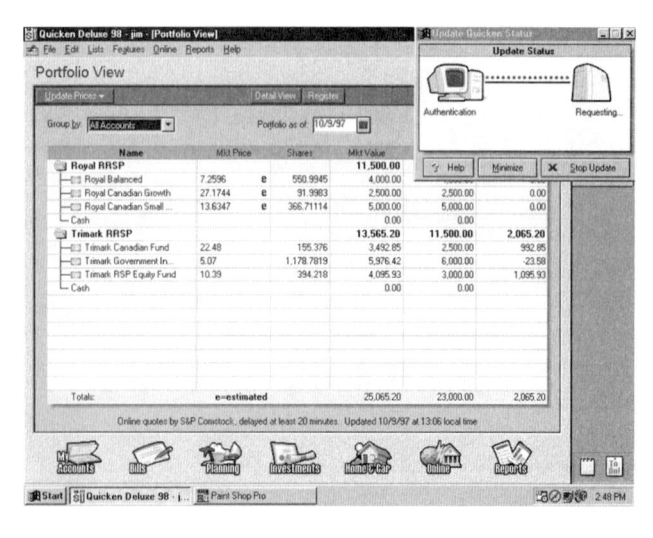

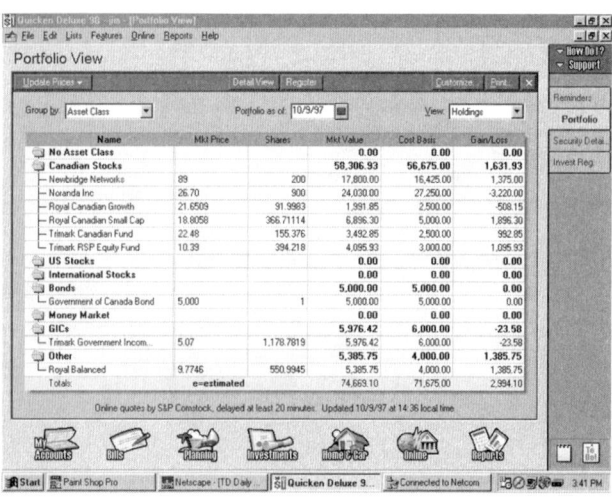

One of the great benefits of the program is that you can generate reports to examine the performance of your investments from a variety of perspectives. You can indicate, for example, what types of information you would like to have appear in your reports:

CHAPTER 9 : Monitoring Your Performance

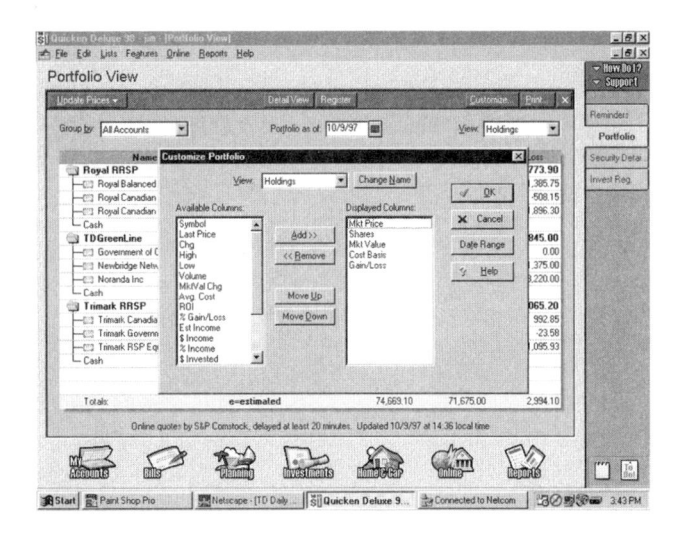

You can choose to view reports about the value of your portfolio, the performance of your investments, how much you have lost or gained once you have sold your investments, or how much income you have made:

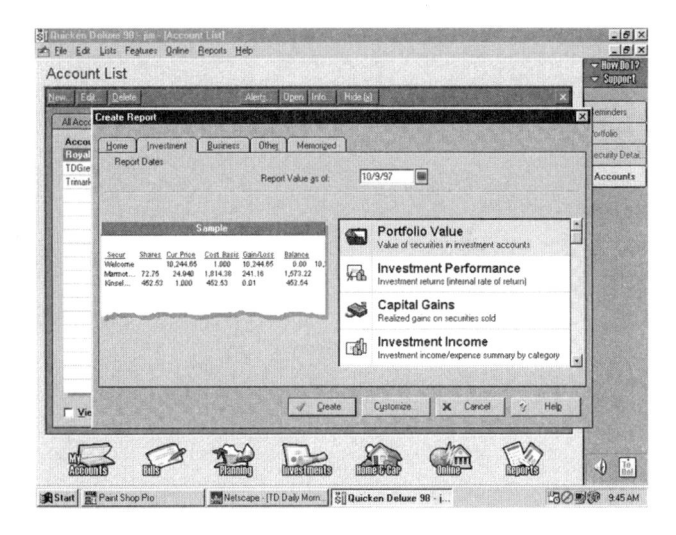

The level of detail and the number of report options are extensive. For example, in the next screen we are examining our performance for the current year, and the report is organized by type of investment. You can also examine this report for any other time period, as seen in the drop-down menu:

1999 MUTUAL FUNDS AND RRSPs ONLINE

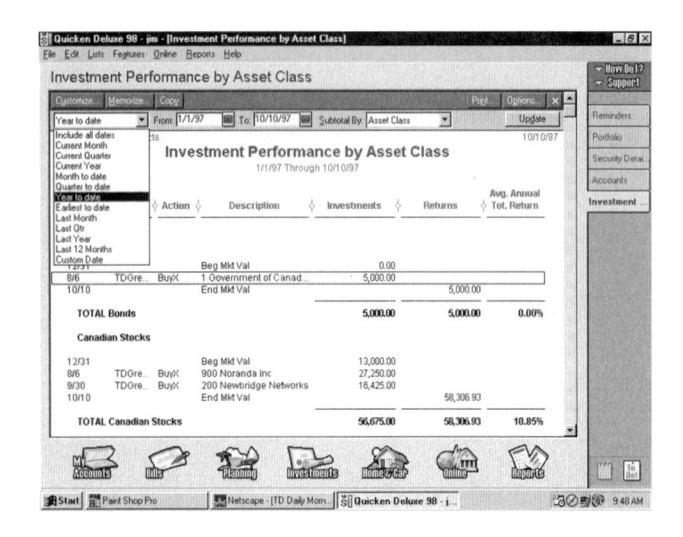

Below, we've asked for a report on our investments, based on our investment objectives. As seen in the drop-down menu, we could view this report in any number of other ways:

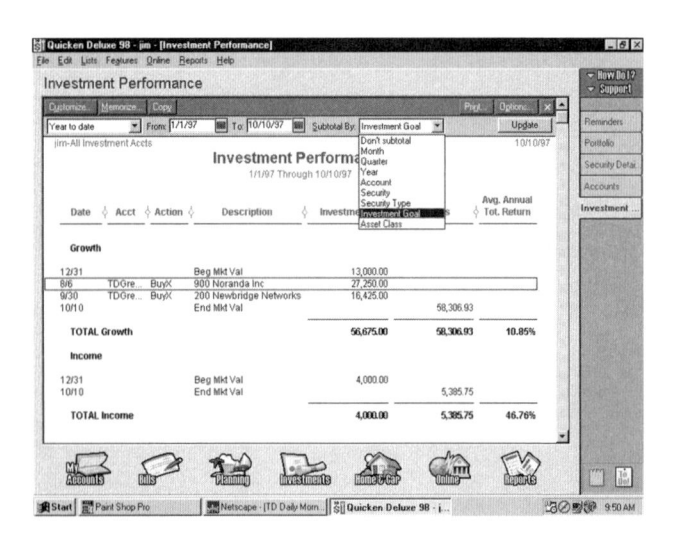

The Bottom Line

It used to be that as an individual investor, unless you had an accounting designation and knew what you were doing, there was very little opportunity for you to easily track the performance of your investments.

This is no longer the case. As we have seen in this chapter, there are many simple but sophisticated and effective tools that you can use to track your investment portfolio. By doing so, you will have a better sense of how you are doing with your investments and a better idea of whether you need to change your approach or objectives.

Web Sites Mentioned in This Chapter

AGF Group of Funds	www.agf.com
Altamira Investment Services	www.altamira.com
Canada Savings Bonds	www.cis-pec.gc.ca
Canada Stockwatch	www.canada-stockwatch.com
Canada Trust	www.canadatrust.com
CANOE	www.canoe.ca
Canadian Stock Market Reporter Inc.	www.canstock.com
Carlson On-line Services Inc.	www.carlsononline.com
Charles Schwab	www.schwab.com
CheckFree Quote Server	www.secapl.com/cgi-bin/qs
CT Securities	www.ctsecurities.com
E*Trade	www.etrade.com
E*Trade Canada	www.canada.etrade.com
freerealtime.com	www.freerealtime.com
The Fund Library	www.fundlibrary.com
GLOBEfund	www.globefund.com
Hepcoe Credit Union	www.hepcoe.com
ilmoney	www.imoney.com
InfoSpace.com	www.infospace.com
Market Guide	www.marketguide.com
Money.com	www.money.com
Munica	www.munica.com
Portfolio Analytics (PALTrak)	www.pal.com
Phillips, Hager & North	www.phn.ca

Quicken.ca	www.quicken.ca
Quote.com	www.quote.com
QuotesCanada.com	www.quotescanada.com
Royal Bank of Canada	www.royalbank.com
Southam Newspapers	www.southam.com
Standard & Poor's	www.personalwealth.com
Stockpoint	www.stockpoint.com
StockSmart	www.stocksmart.com
Telenium	www.telenium.ca
Thomson Real Time Quotes	www.thomsonrtq.com
The Vancouver Sun	www.vancouversun.com

CHAPTER 10

Don't Become Overconfident

Life is a long lesson in humility. JAMES M. BARRIE

HIGHLIGHTS

- **There is a small chorus of voices expressing concern with the concept of online investing.**
- **You should not be overconfident with your use of the Internet, and you should recognize your limitations.**

In the 1980s the popular TV show *Hill Street Blues* featured a police sergeant, who each and every day would say to the officers before they headed out on duty: "And remember, let's be careful out there."

Worthy advice for those of us venturing onto the Internet with our retirement and other investments. And not just because of the fraudulent activities and other problems online that we identified in chapter 2.

We believe that some people might be subjecting themselves to an inordinate degree of risk, because they have become overconfident of their investing abilities as a result of the Internet.

Consider the buzz: the headlines paint the image of how wonderful the world of online investing is. Open any newspaper or magazine, and you see glowing reports on the power to be had through real-time stock quotes, how "now anyone can buy and sell on their own," and how with the arrival of the Internet, you no longer need an investment advisor.

Perhaps a bit of caution is in order when it comes to the hype that surrounds the Internet.

Let us say this: we think that there are tremendous benefits to taking advantage of the investment tools and capabilities on the Internet. At the same time, we fear that some people might go overboard in terms of what they do and in terms of their expectations of their skills.

There are many in the investment world who agree, and they are starting to make their perspectives known.

The Reality?

In an article in the September 23, 1998, edition of the *Wall Street Journal* ("Merrill Says Online Trading is Bad for Investors"), Merrill Lynch Vice Chairman John Steffens stated, quite aggressively, that it was "dangerous" to buy and sell stocks over the Internet.

He wasn't commenting on security issues; rather, he believes that online investing "encourages people to trade too much at the expense of long-term returns." Steffens had been speaking of this perceived risk for some time. He feels that the Internet presents several problems; at one point he compared it to a form of in-home gambling and went so far as to suggest that it can present a serious threat to the financial well-being of investors.

His comments touched off a storm, with critics complaining that Merrill Lynch was simply acting like a "sore loser," because it did not yet have an online brokerage service. There was talk that Merrill was feeling the heat of the lower commission structure of the online world and was concerned that eventually online discount trading would eat into the "fat" commissions it traditionally earned.

> **Charles Schwab, founder of the fast-growing brokerage company, worries about the "2% of investors" who become addicted to the "gambling" aspect found with Internet trading.**

Is such criticism warranted? Much of the buzz surrounding anything to do with the Internet is that it is replacing the "old school" with new methods and new ways of doing business. The perception is that the traditional brokerage business, with its high commissions, is a dinosaur set to be replaced by the invigorating new world of online trading.

But step back from such thinking for a moment, and consider what Steffens was really saying. He was stating a number of concerns, all of which are valid and relate to the fundamental reality that many people might become too cocky with the Internet when it comes to their financial and retirement decisions. Consider the real risks as you explore this online world.

- **You might act short term when you should be thinking long term**

    When it comes to your retirement investments, you should not be subjecting your money to unnecessary high risk by making a lot of short-term decisions. You won't need your RRSP investment for some twenty or thirty or more years. Therefore, many of your investments should be long term in nature. Most investment professionals agree that if you have a long-term investment profile, you shouldn't be doing a lot of trading and selling in the short term.

    The risk of thinking short term with long-term money is particularly true during the current difficult, global investing circumstances. If you listen to the experts, most suggest that we sit tight with our RRSPs, in particular, any stocks that we hold. While prices might be falling fast, tempting you to sell, the fact is that over the longer term the general trend with all equities is upward.

    The problem is that the Internet challenges the long-term line of thinking, in that it makes it all too easy to act in the short term, buying and selling different types of investments. Most professional investors would strongly agree that it is a serious mistake to play on a short-term basis with your long-term money.

- **You might lose the insight and guidance of your investment advisor**

    If you already have an investment counsellor, don't lose sight of his or her role. If you don't have one, maybe you should consider getting one.

Many people might go overboard with the Internet, throwing their investment advisor out the door with a sense of glee. "No more commissions! No more fees! I can do it all on my own!" seems to be the common refrain.

This line of thinking might be a mistake. It's easy to think that with all the information available on the Internet you can "go it alone," make your own financial decisions, and forgo the added expense of professional advice. But for most people that's not a wise move. Professional investment advisors, personal financial planners, and other professionals in the financial industry usually have the expertise, depth of understanding, investment knowledge, and experience that you do not.

The world of finance can be exceedingly complex. Hence, for the average Canadian the Internet should not replace the advice you receive from a professional investment advisor. It's important to keep in mind how an investment professional can help you.

- **You might become overconfident in your abilities**

    It is easy to be in awe of the Internet when it comes to the world of investing: real-time stock quotes, day-to-day portfolio managers, news wires, news updates, all kinds of research reports, and discussion groups that give the "inside scoop."

    We think that there is a risk: not only might people not consider the beneficial role that a traditional investment advisor can play, but they might go overboard in terms of their confidence. All of these high-tech tools are a marvel, and there is a lot we can do online, but overconfidence is dangerous.

The bottom line? When it comes to the world of online investing, recall the story of Icarus, who flew too close to the sun with his wax wings. There is a tremendous opportunity ahead for those of us who take the time to learn to harness the power of the Internet when it comes to our retirement and investment activities.

But if we go overboard, we run the risk of melting our wings.

APPENDIX A

Learning About the Basics of Retirement Planning and RRSPs on the Internet

HIGHLIGHTS

- The Internet is an extremely useful resource for educating yourself on the fundamentals of retirement planning and RRSPs.

- Use caution when accessing RRSP and retirement information on the Internet. Many of the sites are clever sales pitches. We recommend you favour those sites that educate rather than ask for money.

- An integral part of the retirement planning process involves determining how much money you need to save each year in order to retire with a predetermined income in the future.

- An RRSP is the most important retirement vehicle available to Canadians. RRSPs are attractive because most contributions to an RRSP are tax-deductible. In addition, the

> investment income produced by an RRSP is tax-free until you begin to withdraw it.
>
> - Once you retire, you can convert your RRSP into an annuity, a RRIF (a registered retirement income fund), or a life income fund. This allows you to begin using your money upon retirement while minimizing the tax payable on that money.

Retirement Planning

For most people, the words "retirement planning" conjure up the image of running out to the local bank on February 28 to deposit their annual RRSP contribution and figuring out while they're standing in line what type of investment they will place their money into.

But retirement planning is about much more than that; indeed, it is a crucial component of one's financial life. Only by confronting the financial issues of retirement—and understanding why you need to begin saving right away—can you get a full appreciation of the retirement planning process.

There are many questions that you need to ask yourself when you start to plan for your retirement. Sometimes there are so many questions that the process can seem overwhelming and, indeed, almost frightening. But by breaking the process down into several phases you will find that it can become very manageable. The key questions you need to ask yourself are:

- Do I really need to save for my retirement?

- How much am I going to need when I retire?

- How much money do I have now for my retirement, and how much more do I need to save?

- What can I invest in?

- Where do RRSPs fit in? What are some of the key things that I should know about RRSPs?

- What happens to the money I have in my RRSP when I retire?

Fortunately, the Internet has emerged as a tool to help you make your way through the morass of complex RRSP and retirement issues and bring a little excitement to your efforts. It's a veritable gold mine of useful background information that can help you learn more about retirement issues and help you understand the basics of RRSPs.

In this appendix we cover the general aspects of these issues and give a perspective of how you can use the Internet to learn more about many of the specifics related to retirement and RRSPs.

Sales Pitches Online

Of course, there is a double-edged sword at work with the Internet. As useful as this technology is to help learn about retirement planning and RRSPs, you will also discover it to be a cesspool of sales pitches.

Voyage online and you will discover a wealth of advertising, marketing, and sales-oriented material. Each and every investment site seems to offer its own definitive theory about how Canadians should invest for their retirement. All too often, a company will suggest that the magic solution to your retirement planning needs is simply to buy a particular mutual fund that they happen to sell.

Your challenge in using the Internet is to sift through the vast amounts of sales-oriented information and find the useful stuff.

That is where this appendix will come in handy. We offer some guidance on what you should be looking for, and where you should be looking, in order to get useful retirement- and RRSP-related information.

Do I Really Need to Save for My Retirement?

Yes you do.

If you have a job, you can't expect your company's pension plan or the Canada Pension Plan to necessarily provide you with enough income upon retirement. In fact, these sources might very well be inadequate to give you the income necessary to meet your retirement expectations. Further, given some estimates that many people will find themselves working in as many as six to eight different jobs in their lifetime, it is likely that many people won't have one good, long-term corporate pension plan to take care of them in the future.

If you are self-employed, as many Canadians are, the situation is even more dramatic: you are solely responsible for taking care of yourself in retirement, since there isn't any company pension plan whatsoever.

There are some Web sites that provide information about retirement and financial planning concepts but aren't affiliated with any particular financial organization. This makes them a good source for independent information.

One of the best examples is RetireWeb, a resource that provides a good, concise overview of the retirement planning process. The authors of the site suggest that you spend a good five hours reading the information and using the tools they make available.

The site provides useful background information about what you can expect from the government upon retirement as well as pointers to documents that describe the crisis within the Canadian pension system. It also includes a glossary if you run into retirement or financial terms you don't understand.

We do have concerns with how frequently the site is updated. When we visited, it hadn't been updated for some time, so you should take care to ensure that any information that it provides is up-to-date:

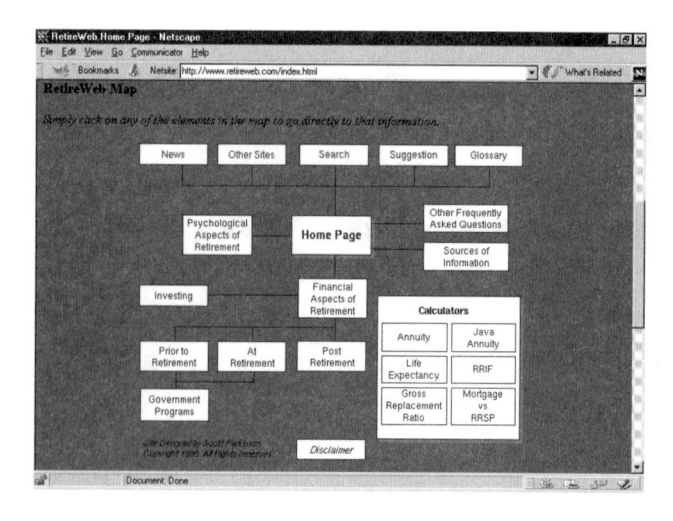

APPENDIX A: Learning About the Basics of Retirement Planning and RRSPs on the Internet

What if you have retired already or are about to and need specific retirement information such as what payments you can expect from the government?

Take a look at the Seniors Computer Information Project. This is an initiative set up to help senior citizens access online information resources, and it features the Manitoba Senior Citizens Handbook, which includes a lengthy overview of the financial benefits that can be expected upon retirement. It is one of the best online sources for basic information about the Canada Pension Plan and other government income sources:

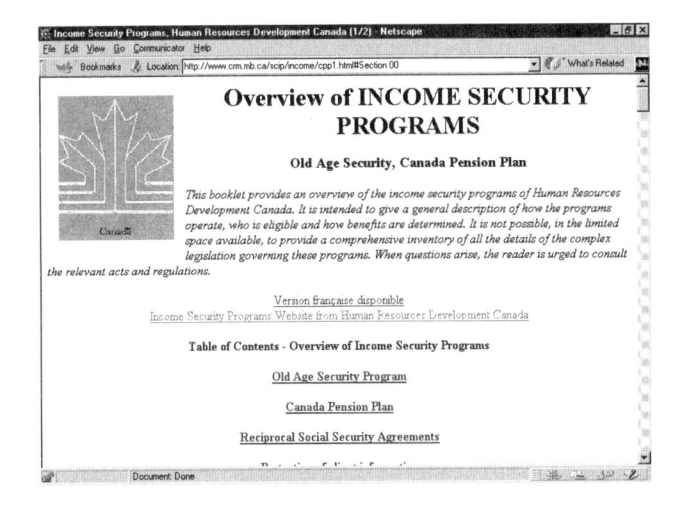

With so much focus on the CPP and its ability (or inability) to make payments in the future, you might expect the Canadian government to offer a useful online guide about retirement planning. But at the time this book went to press, we couldn't find one; information seems to be scattered here and there. Revenue Canada maintains a Web site with answers to questions about retirement/RRSP issues as they relate to taxes, but it's not an easy site to use, nor does it contain a lot of useful information.

You can visit the official Canada Pension Plan site, but it seems more oriented toward informing you about how the Canadian pension system will be overhauled.

Finally, go to the Human Resources Development Canada Web site, and you will find some useful information under the Income Security Programs section. The site has been recently redesigned to make it more user friendly.

How Much Am I Going to Need When I Retire?

Many Canadians think that their company pension plan will be sufficient for their retirement years. But once they look into these pension plans they often discover that the payments upon retirement are not what they thought.

Not only that, but there is some risk attached to corporate pension plans: there have been a few situations involving the failure of a corporate plan and situations in which a plan had insufficient funds to pay what was promised. What guarantee do you have that a company pension plan will be able to meet all of its obligations in the future?

In addition to this, many Canadians have come to realize that Canada's social programs will not allow them, when they retire, to maintain the lifestyle they have become accustomed to.

For a long time Canada has lived with the philosophy that the government is responsible for ensuring that Canadians have enough retirement income. The CPP was established in 1966, and its founding principles still stand: every employed and self-employed person working in Canada contributes to the plan, and both they and their family members are eligible to receive payment from the plan in case of retirement, disability, or death.

But the government's "social safety net" doesn't provide much money: the CPP provides payments of less than $15,000 per annum to those who were gainfully employed. Another plan, the government Old Age Security system, provides less than $5,000 per annum to most Canadian citizens over the age of 65.

Having reviewed these two issues you may find that you alone are responsible for your future financial circumstances.

Obviously, once you retire, you will no longer have a salary, but you will still need money to pay for your day-to-day living expenses. In addition to that, you might need money to travel, to help out family members, or even to purchase a retirement home in Florida or elsewhere if you are so inclined.

APPENDIX A: Learning About the Basics of Retirement Planning and RRSPs on the Internet

How do you go about figuring out how much money you will need to save to retire? First, figure out what you spend your money on today, and then decide if that is how you will spend your money when you retire. You should think about how much you spend each month, for example:

- **Mortgage/Rent payments.** Do you make these payments now? Do you think you will have to make them when you retire, or will you be self-sufficient in terms of home ownership? How much money will you need to cover any future nursing home expenses?

- **Living expenses.** What do you spend today on clothing, food, utilities, automobiles, and other necessities? What will you expect to spend upon retirement?

- **Family expenses.** Do you support any children? Will the children be finished their education by the time you retire, or will you be supporting them? Do you think you will have to support any other family members when you retire?

- **Entertainment and travel expenses.** Do you plan to travel when you retire? If so, how much do you want to have available for such discretionary expenses in the future?

These are only a few examples of what you will need to consider when you determine how much money you will need per year when you retire. You have to give a lot of thought to where you will be spending money some twenty, thirty, or forty years from now to get a rough idea of the annual income that you will need.

And just to compound the matter, the yearly income amount that you will be calculating is based on today's dollar. To properly figure out your required annual income on retirement, you will need to consider inflation in your calculations.

What should you do? Sit down with pen and paper—or a spreadsheet—and roughly work out the annual income you expect to require upon retirement, based on what you are spending today and what you will spend in the future.

1999 MUTUAL FUNDS AND RRSPs ONLINE

There are tools on the Internet that can help you do this, such as this spreadsheet on the Web site of First Canadian Mutual Funds, the mutual funds arm of the Bank of Montreal:

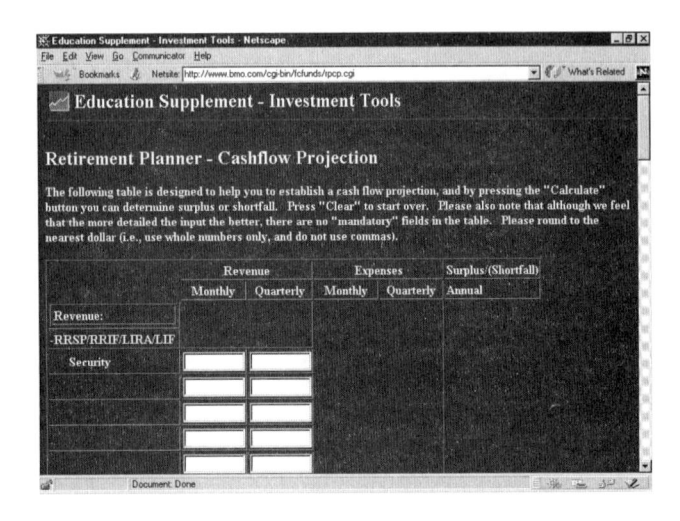

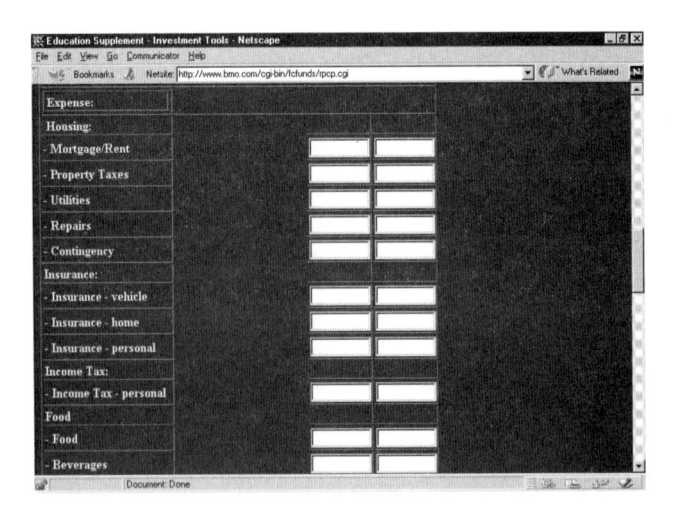

How Much Money Do I Have Now for My Retirement, and How Much More Do I Need to Save?

Having figured out how much you will need to retire, the next question is knowing how much you will need to save in order to achieve that goal.

APPENDIX A: Learning About the Basics of Retirement Planning and RRSPs on the Internet

No matter what the amount, you have to begin saving today. To have a secure financial future upon retirement, you will have to have put away a sum of money this and each year leading up to your retirement, in order to supplement any funds that will be available from your pension plan and from the CPP. The money that you save will then be used to provide your desired retirement "salary" for the remaining years of your life.

Of course, to figure out how much you need to save every year, you must answer two of the hardest questions when it comes to retirement planning:

- What annual income will you need throughout your retirement?

- How long do you expect to live after you retire?

The complexity doesn't stop here. There are other factors that will affect how much you need to save. For example, at what age do you plan to retire? There can be a big difference between the amount you must save each year if you plan to retire at the age of 55 instead of 65.

Let's put all of this into perspective using a simplified example and the "Retirement Planning Calculator" found on the TDBank Web site. Let's say you plan to retire early, at the age of 60, and figure you will live to the ripe old age of 80. You'd like to have an annual income each year of $50,000, figuring that will be enough to take care of your needs, based on the work that you did as we described above. Today you are 35 years old:

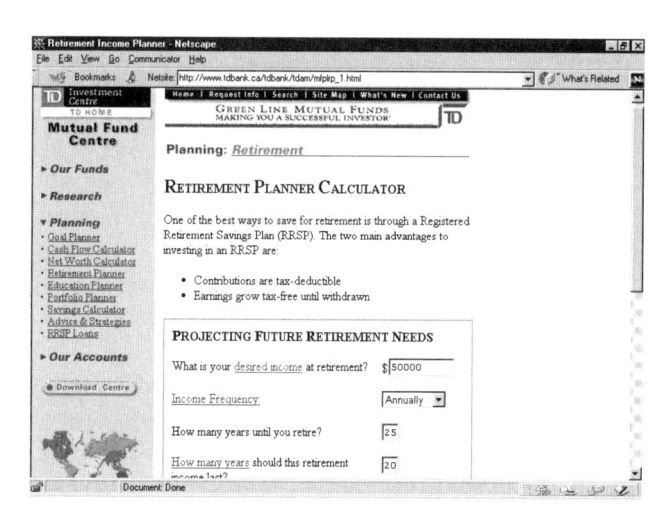

Using these types of tools helps us to factor in the "time value of money." This means that we can indicate what we think the inflation rate will be in the future as well as what we think our investments will earn. If we assume a 3% inflation rate and a 10% rate of return on our investments, the amount we will need to invest every year will be $8,761.47:

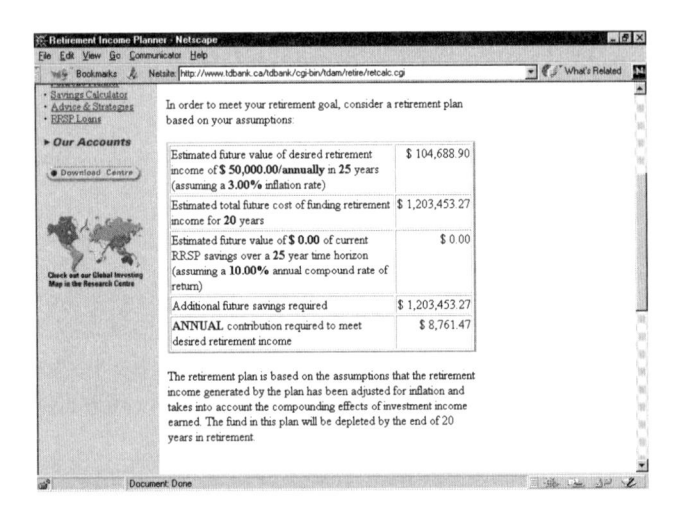

[Screenshot: Retirement Income Planner - Netscape]

Estimated future value of desired retirement income of **$ 50,000.00/annually** in 25 years (assuming a **3.00%** inflation rate)	$ 104,688.90
Estimated total future cost of funding retirement income for **20 years**	$ 1,203,453.27
Estimated future value of **$ 0.00** of current RRSP savings over a **25 year** time horizon (assuming a **10.00%** annual compound rate of return)	$ 0.00
Additional future savings required	$ 1,203,453.27
ANNUAL contribution required to meet desired retirement income	$ 8,761.47

The retirement plan is based on the assumptions that the retirement income generated by the plan has been adjusted for inflation and takes into account the compounding effects of investment income earned. The fund in this plan will be depleted by the end of 20 years in retirement.

There are a number of online calculators that take into account this time value of money in their estimation of what you must save each year. Many of these calculators also take into consideration any RRSP savings that you already have, any income that you receive from a company pension plan if you have one, or the CPP, helping you come up with a more accurate calculation of how much you need to save each year.

Understanding Your Current Coverage

Don't forget where your company pension plan fits into this whole situation. Money that is invested in your company pension plan is also compounding, and your company pension representatives can give you a good idea of what type of payment you can expect during your retirement as a result.

So if you are employed and your company has a pension plan—and this is important—you should definitely consider taking part. In addition, ask your company pension representative for a clear calculation of the benefits you will receive upon retirement. Make sure you understand what the benefits would be if you decided to retire early. Finally, ask if you are currently taking advantage of maximum contributions; you may not be. If not, find out how to do so and whether you can make "prior-year catch-up payments" in order to ensure that you have contributed the maximum amount for all prior years.

You should also determine what you will get from the CPP, keeping in mind that you may not see some of this money, since it could be "clawed back" through your income tax return. (There is a lot of talk that as the CPP system is restructured, those in a high income bracket upon retirement will have to "pay back" the CPP payments they have received; this is often referred to as a "claw back.")

Take some time to understand what monthly or annual payment you will get from these two sources upon retirement. This will help you when using the online tools to more accurately calculate what your savings requirements will be.

What Can I Invest In?

After you complete these calculations, you will likely be shocked at the amount you need to save to fund your retirement expectations. For many people it will not be easy to save $12,000 or so per year for their retirement.

In order to work out a plan to accomplish your objectives, there are two important issues that you must address:

- how you will save the money necessary for your retirement, and

- what kinds of investments will provide a suitable return to help ensure that your money grows.

The first issue can be a pretty serious challenge for many people, and there is not much advice we can give on what to do. If you don't have any extra money that you can save and things are pretty tight, you must simply decide that saving for your retirement is something that you really want to do and that you will work hard to accomplish it. This means cutting back current expenses and juggling your current financial situation; it could mean that you have a lot of work to do to improve your current financial circumstances.

The investment issue is more straightforward. The types of investments are endless: bonds, guaranteed investment certificates (GICs), Canada Savings Bonds (CSBs), common and preferred shares, real estate, mutual funds, etc. For many the primary retirement investment consists of the value of the home, given the likelihood that it will be mortgage-free upon retirement and can be sold for a profit (assuming there is someplace else to move to).

There are many Web sites that provide information on the different types of investments you can hold defining the risks and benefits of each. One such site is the i|money Web site:

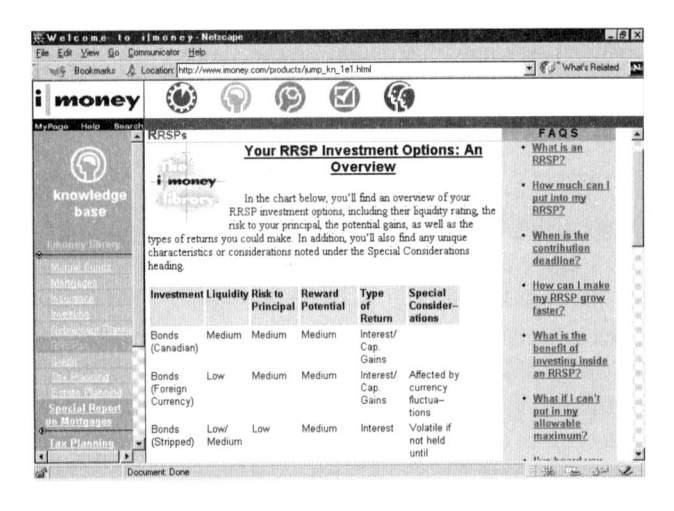

Where Do RRSPs Fit In? What Are Some of the Key Things I Should Know About RRSPs?

Some time ago the federal government established the Registered Retirement Savings Plan (RRSP) when it realized that it would be in its best interest to encourage Canadians to save for their retirement.

An RRSP is essentially a retirement investment, made under very stringent rules, that provides a tax deduction equal to the amount of the investment. The amount that you can invest depends on your particular situation. Making the maximum RRSP contribution that you can each year is probably one of the smartest financial moves that you can undertake.

What Are the Advantages of Having an RRSP?

There are two main tax advantages to investing in an RRSP:

- The amount you contribute is usually deductible on your tax return, making the RRSP one of the last remaining "tax loopholes" with which to reduce your income tax.

- The income earned in an RRSP is tax-free until you withdraw the funds, either as a lump sum or in regular withdrawals, for example, yearly, quarterly, monthly, upon retirement.

What an RRSP lets you do, in essence, is obtain "free money" from the government. What do you do to get this free money? You promise to put away your own money and not touch it until your retirement.

The amount of tax that you can save by investing money in an RRSP can be dramatic, depending on your level of income and, hence, the tax bracket or "marginal tax rate" that you fall into.

What Are Some of the Key Things to Know?

There are many questions that surround RRSPs and retirement information. Here are just a few of the questions you need to answer:

- What are the differences between nondirected and self-directed RRSPs?

- What is my marginal tax rate, and how does it affect my RRSP?

- What types of investments can I hold in my RRSP?

- Is an RRSP protected if the organization in which the investment is held collapses?

- How much should/could I put into my RRSP?

- Should I put money into my RRSP or pay down my mortgage?

- Does it make sense to borrow to make my RRSP contribution?

- What is a spousal RRSP?

- What happens if I need money?

There are several places on the Internet that can help you find the answers to these and many other questions, for example, the Web sites run by major newspapers and magazines.

These sites are particularly useful during RRSP season—January and February—when most publications generate a flood of material devoted to the topic. Fortunately, many publications do not remove their RRSP articles once the season has ended, recognizing that they are of benefit long after the primary RRSP season is finished.

A number of publications have taken previously published articles and used them to create special financial sections on their Web sites. These collections are an excellent source of independent financial advice.

For example, *The Ottawa Citizen* Web site features articles and commentary about RRSPs in the Your Money and Business sections. It is an excellent starting point:

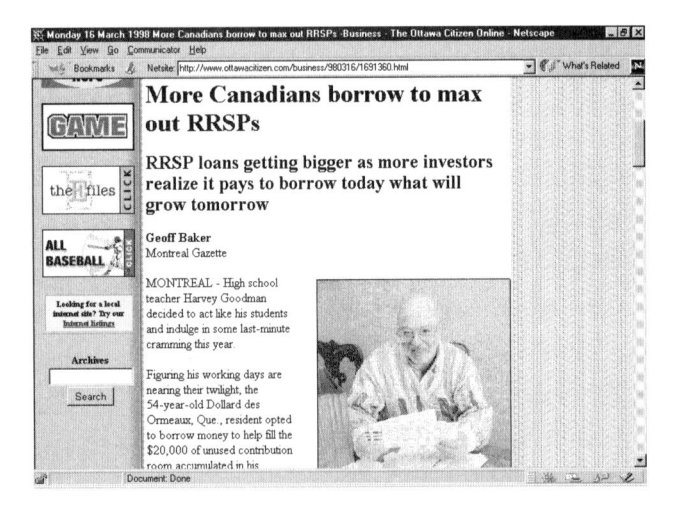

And you can check out GLOBEfund, from the *Globe and Mail*. Although oriented toward mutual funds, its education centre does feature some retirement information:

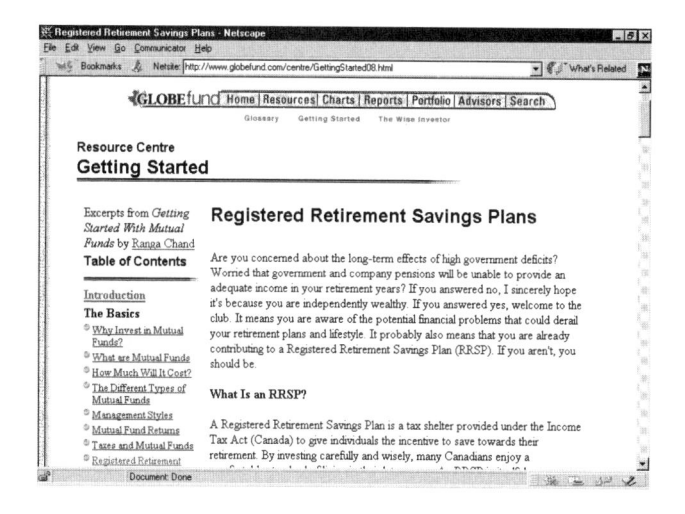

APPENDIX A: Learning About the Basics of Retirement Planning and RRSPs on the Internet

There are several Canadian financial magazines with Web sites, but we have found them sadly lacking in terms of online content. Two notable examples that cover retirement/RRSP issues in print are the *All-Canadian Mutual Fund Guide* and *IE:Money,* the latter having much useful information online:

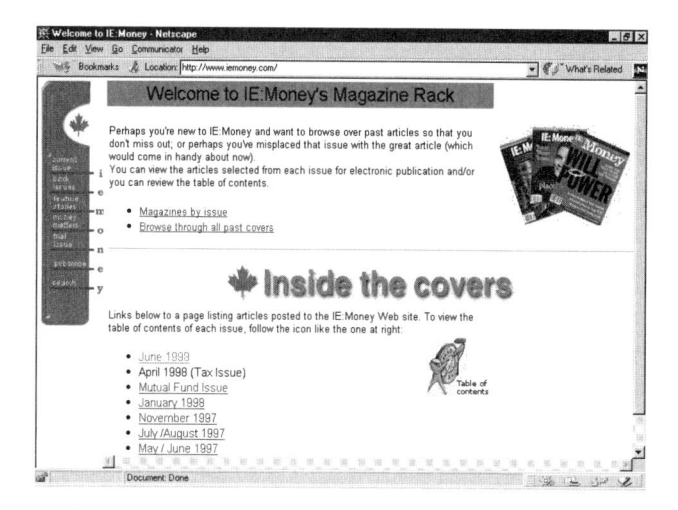

In addition, take a look at the Retirement Planning Section of Quicken.ca and the Retirement section of the i|money Knowledge Base.

Also check out the Web sites of accounting firms. You will find that many small, regional accounting firms and some of the "big five" accounting firms (Arthur

Andersen, KPMG, Deloitte & Touche, Ernst & Young, PricewaterhouseCoopers) offer tax information on their Web sites, which sometimes includes details about RRSPs and retirement.

This information is often available in the newsletters that these organizations publish online or in specially designed "RRSP centres." Because such firms are not actively involved in the sale of financial products, but limit their activities to the provision of financial advice, the information they offer is independent.

One of the best online services offered by one of the big accounting firms in Canada, Ernst & Young, is their "tax mailbag" feature. On their Web site tax professionals respond to questions submitted by Internet users, and the answers are published so that everyone can benefit from the responses. Since many of the questions pertain to RRSPs and retirement planning, it is an excellent source of free but valuable information. They also include a calculator that estimates your tax savings generated by your RRSP contribution:

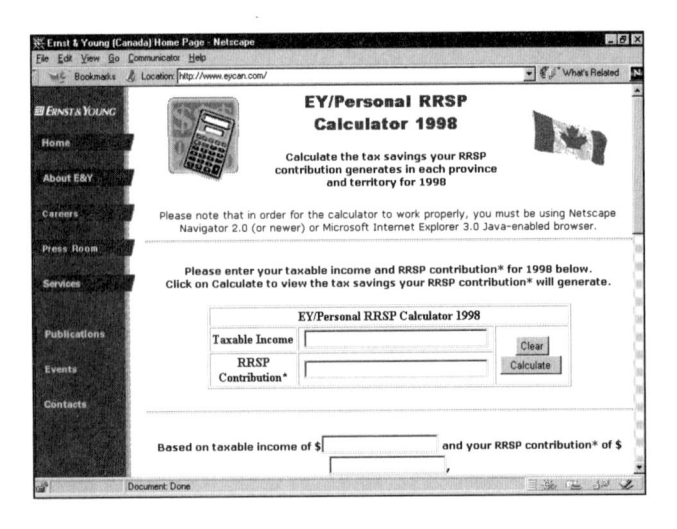

However, despite the foregoing, as with newspapers and magazines, you will find many of the accounting firm sites to be lacking in useful content.

You can also find retirement information on the Web sites of many professional financial planners and advisors.

Since many of these operations are small, one-person organizations, you will find that their Web sites are often

APPENDIX A: Learning About the Basics of Retirement Planning and RRSPs on the Internet

limited in the scope of information they offer. Indeed, it seems that the number of planners and professional advisors who provide truly useful retirement information online is rather limited; we haven't found many that have good, compelling, useful background information with respect to retirement/RRSP issues.

When you do find a site that provides some information, remember that many financial planners represent certain mutual fund or other financial organizations and are directly involved in the sale of such products. Given that their income is most often generated on a commission or similar basis, the advice they offer is not necessarily independent or unbiased.

Where else should you look? Many financial authors and journalists have set up their own Web sites to disseminate investment information. For example, Gordon Pape, a well-known Canadian financial expert, has his own Web site. You can often find useful retirement/RRSP-related information there and in other similar sites.

What Happens to the Money I Have in My RRSP When I Retire?

You have three choices, each of which must be carried out by December 31 of the year you turn 69:

- You can withdraw all the money from the RRSP and pay tax on it immediately. Not a terribly good idea, since much of the money will be taxed at the highest possible tax rate, which could mean that you could immediately lose half of your total RRSP investment!

- Move the money into an "annuity" (which you can actually do before the age of 69) so that you withdraw the money gradually throughout your retirement. This ensures that much of the money in your RRSP is taxed at the lowest possible tax rate; since there is a tiered tax rate system in Canada, you want to ensure that you get as much income as you can, taxed at the lowest possible rate. This can be accomplished by spreading your RRSP money out over a number of years.

- Move the money into a Registered Retirement Income Fund (RRIF), which is like an annuity but has some special features that make it more attractive.

Clearly, you have to decide between choosing an annuity and a RRIF.

Annuities are most often sold by insurance and trust companies. An annuity is an investment that pays a sum of money on a regular basis, usually every month, over a fixed period of time, such as ten years. This allows you to receive the money from your RRSP investment over a period of time, spreading out the tax bill on this money. Income earned on the money in the annuity is subject to tax as it is earned. Once you purchase an annuity, your control of how the money is invested ends; it is left up to the company that you purchased the annuity from to decide how to invest it. Also, unless you buy an indexed annuity, the amount of your monthly payment will be the same year after year, regardless of inflation or any changes in your financial needs.

A RRIF is like an annuity in that you are provided a regular stream of payments, thereby spreading the tax bill over several years. However, unlike an annuity, the income earned on the money in the RRIF is accumulated tax-free. As some have said, a RRIF is like an RRSP in reverse, since the money earned in the RRIF is tax-free and instead of contributing over time, you are withdrawing over time. Another key difference between an annuity and a RRIF is that with a RRIF you determine what you wish to invest in, much as you do with your RRSP. Another important aspect of a RRIF is that you must withdraw a certain amount each year, ranging from 7% to 9%, depending on your age.

Obviously, a RRIF will make sense for most people given that the income in it accumulates tax-free. Again, there are many places on the Internet that can give you guidance on what annuities and RRIFs are and how to deal with them. The Fund Library is one such site:

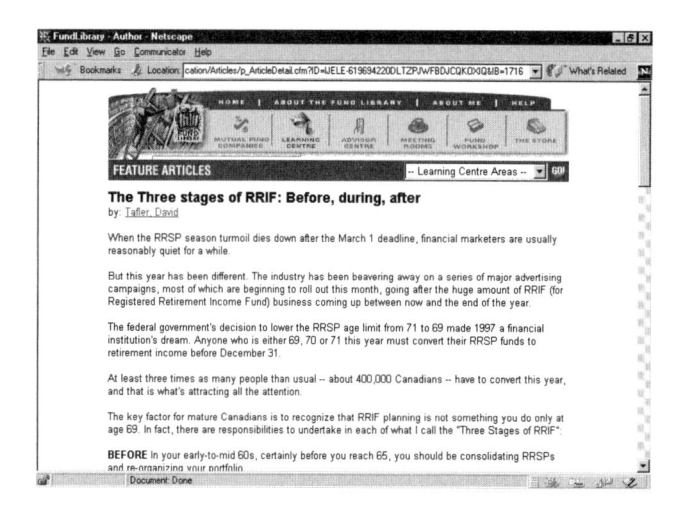

APPENDIX A: Learning About the Basics of Retirement Planning and RRSPs on the Internet

> **FEATURE ARTICLES**
>
> **The Three stages of RRIF: Before, during, after**
> by: Tafler, David
>
> When the RRSP season turmoil dies down after the March 1 deadline, financial marketers are usually reasonably quiet for a while.
>
> But this year has been different. The industry has been beavering away on a series of major advertising campaigns, most of which are beginning to roll out this month, going after the huge amount of RRIF (for Registered Retirement Income Fund) business coming up between now and the end of the year.
>
> The federal government's decision to lower the RRSP age limit from 71 to 69 made 1997 a financial institution's dream. Anyone who is either 69, 70 or 71 this year must convert their RRSP funds to retirement income before December 31.
>
> At least three times as many people than usual -- about 400,000 Canadians -- have to convert this year, and that is what's attracting all the attention.
>
> The key factor for mature Canadians is to recognize that RRIF planning is not something you do only at age 69. In fact, there are responsibilities to undertake in each of what I call the "Three Stages of RRIF":
>
> **BEFORE** In your early-to-mid 60s, certainly before you reach 65, you should be consolidating RRSPs and re-organizing your portfolio.

Summary

When using the Internet to learn about RRSP and retirement issues, we suggest you use those sites that educate rather than those sites that focus on the hard sell. It is hard enough to try to get a good understanding of retirement and RRSP issues without trying to figure out what retirement products are the best suited to your particular circumstances.

Here are five tips to help you when looking for retirement and/or RRSP information on the Internet:

- **Constantly revisit sites**

  Web sites change constantly. Revisit sites on a regular basis to see what's new.

- **Learn to distinguish useful content from a sales pitch**

  Look for the sites that take the time to answer your questions, rather than the sites that seem to want to sell you something. As you use the Internet, you'll come to recognize the difference between the two approaches.

- **Look for a FAQ**

  Many sites with useful content provide a retirement or RRSP FAQ. This is a summary of answers to "frequently asked questions" and is an excellent place to start.

- **Complement the information**

    The information you obtain from the Web sites of banks, mutual fund companies, and insurance companies should be complemented with independent sources of information such as articles and reports from newspapers, magazines, and accounting/consulting organizations.

- **Question the information**

    Check any information you obtain from the Internet. Many online publications and newsletters are sponsored by companies or individuals with a direct involvement in the sales of products mentioned in the publication.

Web Sites Mentioned in This Appendix

All-Canadian Mutual Fund Guide	www.mutualfundguide-ca.com
Arthur Andersen Canada	www.arthurandersen/canada/index.asp
Canada Pension Plan	www.cpp-rpc.gc.ca
Deloitte & Touche Canada	www.deloitte.ca
Ernst & Young Canada	www.eycan.com
First Canadian Mutual Funds	www.bmo.com/fcfunds
The Fund Library	www.fundlibrary.com
GLOBEfund	www.globefund.com
Gordon Pape	www.gordonpape.com
Human Resources Development Canada	www.hrdc-drhc.gc.ca
IE:Money	www.iemoney.com
ilmoney	www.imoney.com
KPMG Canada	www.kpmg.ca
The Ottawa Citizen	www.ottawacitizen.com
PricewaterhouseCoopers Canada	www.pwcglobal.com/ca
Quicken.ca	www.quicken.ca
RetireWeb	www.retireweb.com

APPENDIX A: Learning About the Basics of Retirement Planning and RRSPs on the Internet

Revenue Canada	www.rc.gc.ca
Seniors Computer Information Project	www.crm.mb.ca/scip
TD Bank	www.tdbank.ca

APPENDIX B

Basic Investment Concepts

HIGHLIGHTS

- In order to determine what types of investments you want to place your money in, you need to understand your financial objectives, your risk tolerance level, and whether you are an active or passive investor.

- Assessing a financial investment involves examining its income, growth, and risk characteristics. Every investment can be evaluated on these three important criteria.

- Most investments fall into one of three basic categories: cash-based (for example, savings accounts), debt (for example, bonds), and equity (for example, stocks).

Whether you intend to place your RRSP money into an investment such as a mutual fund that is managed by someone else or establish a self-directed RRSP so that you can more closely and directly manage your own investments, you will need to have an understanding of the types of financial investments that are available and appropriate for you. After determining your financial goals, one of the first steps is considering the type of risk that you are willing to accept with your investments.

This isn't an easy thing to do. Determining what kinds of investments to make can be quite a challenge. The Internet can aid you greatly in this regard. If you learn to use it properly, it will help you with your investment decisions. But by the same token, if you don't fully comprehend what you are trying to accomplish before getting online, the Internet can confuse you greatly or cause you to make poor financial decisions.

That's why we've written this appendix, to review basic investment concepts so that you have a solid grounding in these issues *before* you plunge into the vast array of financial resources that are available online. This appendix discusses two important concepts:

- the type of investor you are; and
- the types of investments that are available.

Do You Know What Type of Investor You Are?

Many Canadians do not invest in anything other than savings accounts, Canada Savings Bonds, or mutual funds. Even when they place their money in these types of investments, they often haven't taken the time to consider why they chose a particular investment or the type of return that they might earn on such an investment. In addition, many Canadians give little thought to the risk associated with the investments they've chosen.

What is the reason for this? From our research we get the feeling that many people have an overwhelming sense that the world of finance is too complex for them to comprehend. And there is no doubt that there is inertia at work here. Many people simply don't take the time to learn about investing, and as a result, take the easy way out by choosing an investment that offers the least amount of complexity. Hence, every year around February 28, Canadians rush to buy mutual funds without really thinking about what they are doing.

Intelligent RRSP decisions involve more than simply grabbing the first uncomplicated financial investment that's put in front of you. To really know what you are doing, you have to understand the types of investments that are available to you. But even before you consider specific types of investments, you need to know what type of investor you are.

Income, Growth, and Risk

When it comes to making an investment, the trick to deciding where to place your money is to determine the types of investments that you feel the most comfortable with. To figure this out, you need to consider the growth and income potential of your investments as well as the risk of the various investments you place your money into.

Any investment that you make will offer a potential return. You will see the value of the investment grow (such as increase in the stock price), and you might earn income on the investment (such as interest on a bond). Some investments will offer both growth potential and income (such as dividend-paying stocks), others will offer only income (as with a term deposit), and yet others will offer only the potential for growth (gold, for example).

But investments are characterized not only by their growth potential or the income they generate. They also carry a certain degree of risk.

When it comes to risk, there is a general rule of thumb that applies to investing. Low-risk investments usually offer fairly low returns. Investments that are riskier generally offer high returns. Hence, if you want high returns, you usually have to be willing to accept high risk.

Figuring out what types of investments you are most comfortable with requires an understanding of your risk tolerance level—simply, how much risk you are willing to put up with when it comes to your investments. The higher your risk tolerance level, the more risk you are willing to take.

For some people, the thought of holding an investment where they might see significant growth but where they have an equal chance of losing 30% or more of their money causes many sleepless nights. But for other people, this is quite an acceptable level of risk, and necessary to obtain a higher return on their investment. You need to find what level of risk you are comfortable with before you start investing.

There are many articles and newsletters in financial magazines and newspapers that discuss the concept of risk. In addition, many financial organizations have designed questionnaires that you can fill out to help you understand where you fall on the "risk scale." Determining the extent of risk that you are willing to tolerate really comes down to doing some creative thinking on your part, as well as thoroughly examining your own particular financial circumstances and investment attitudes.

Ultimately, when you assess a particular investment you need to think about its growth, income, and risk characteristics, and whether these factors fit your investment goals.

Diversify!

Once you have determined the level of risk that you are willing to tolerate, the next step is to put together a long-term investment strategy.

It is important to keep in mind that when it comes to investing for your retirement, your strategy is for the long term. After all, you will be putting money away for ten, twenty, or thirty years or more.

It may sound complicated to put together an investment strategy, but it really isn't. If you decide that you are at the low end of the risk scale, that is, you don't want to tolerate a high amount of risk, then your strategy for investing should be to find very stable, guaranteed types of investments. These investments offer little risk but steady income and/or growth. If you find you are at the high end of the risk scale, and you are willing to take a chance on losing some of your investment money, your strategy should be to find investments that have high growth and income potential.

Regardless of where you are on the risk scale, you should always invest in more than one type of investment. This is called diversifying your portfolio—you might consider placing some of your money in a high-risk investment to achieve some growth and part of it in low-risk investments to ensure stability in the value of your investment.

Putting all your money into low-risk investments may let you sleep at night, but your investment may not grow enough over the long term to give you the level of income that you will need to retire with. Conversely, investing in only high-risk items may give you high growth and income potential, but you may lose a substantial amount of your investment if a few investments fail. This is another way of saying "don't put all your eggs in one basket." You want to be able to spread your money over different types of investments so that you can achieve the growth you need and the retirement income you desire.

Once you have decided on a long-term strategy (that is, what percentage of your investments will be low, medium, and high risk), stick to it!

Remember that your strategy is for the *long term*. You might not see results with a particular investment right away. And given the constant fluctuation in such areas as the stock market and the price of gold, there will be ups and downs along the way. But it is the cumulative effect that you need to pay attention to. For example, over the long term, the values of investments on the stock market have risen, even though there were substantial decreases in 1987 and in the early 1990s.

Understand What You Are Investing In

One final thing before we go into detail about the types of investments to consider. Make sure you understand what you are investing in *before* you invest.

This may sound like a silly statement, but a lot of people are guilty of not doing this. How many times have you gone to the bank on February 28 to make your RRSP contribution, only to have the bank manager inform you of some new investment opportunities? Then she asks you why you're not taking advantage of the foreign content rules.

There you sit, stumped! Here you thought you had figured out what you were going to invest in, and suddenly you find yourself grabbing the first RRSP investment she pushes at you.

It will do you a lot of good to do some research beforehand to understand the types of investments you should be considering. For one thing, you will be able to assess the new financial products that come onto the market every year and determine if they are right for you. Second, you will be able to ask the right questions about these new products when talking to your bank manager or financial professional. Questions such as:

- What is the risk of that investment?

- What is its growth potential?

- Is there any guarantee on the value of the investment?

- Is it covered by any type of deposit or other form of insurance?
- What is the growth and income history of the investment?

What Type of Investor Are You?

One important outcome of this preparatory work is that you will begin to understand whether you are an active or passive investor.

An active investor is an individual who takes great delight in tracking the value and activity of his or her investment portfolio on a daily basis and enjoys tracking stock markets, financial news, and other information.

A passive investor, on the other hand, is an individual who doesn't have the time or inclination to track each and every investment on a day-to-day basis, and takes little joy in the whole activity of investing and finance.

It is fair to say that your investment decisions with respect to growth, income, and risk will probably be reflected in the type of investor you are. If you have the time, interest, and passion to track your investments on a regular basis, you will probably also be more interested in investments that offer a little more growth yet bear more risk. In comparison, investors who can't afford the time to track their own investments will usually be interested in investments that are more conservative.

Types of Financial Investments

Once you have put together your long-term investment strategy, assessed your risk level, and determined what type of investor you are, it is time to find the investments that are right for you.

When it comes right down to it, there are essentially three types of investments that you can make: cash-based, debt, and equity.

- **Cash-based**
  Your investment is a form of cash, such as a savings account or GIC.

- **Debt**
  You invest in the debt issued by an organization, such as a bond. Your income is derived from the interest that the organization pays on that debt as well as any gain or loss in the underlying value of the debt. It is important to keep in mind that the overall value of a bond fluctuates on financial markets just as stock prices do—even though a bond might be issued for $1,000, its value on the market can range above or below this amount before its due date (also referred to as "maturity"). On its due date it will be worth exactly $1,000.

- **Equity**
  You invest in some type of ownership in the organization. Your income is derived from the increase in the overall worth of the organization as well as from the payment of income (usually in the form of a dividend) on the investment.

The financial world has dreamed up all kinds of hybrids of these three basic options, but for simplicity's sake, anything you invest in fits into one of these three basic categories.

Every investment has three basic characteristics that we described earlier: income, growth potential, and risk.

- **Income**
  The amount of income produced by the investment. Income is often in the form of interest or dividends.

- **Growth potential**
  This is the amount that the investment increases or decreases in overall value in addition to any income earned. The growth potential might range from low to high to aggressive. The larger the growth potential, the higher the potential risk of the investment.

- **Risk**
  Some investments are riskier than others by being more prone to loss. This loss may occur in several ways. For example, the investment may decrease in value (such as might happen with a stock). Alternatively, you could lose the full value of the investment (such as might happen with your shares in a company that goes bankrupt or collapses in value).

The following table can be used as a rough guide to the income, growth potential, and risk associated with the various types of investments that we discussed in this book.

Investment	Income	Growth Potential	Risk
Savings account	Low	Low	Low
Canada Savings Bonds (CSBs)	Medium	Low	Low
Term Deposits/ Guaranteed Investment Certificates (GICs)	Medium	Low	Low/Medium
Preferred shares	Medium	Low	Medium
Common shares	Low/Medium	High	Medium/High
Bonds	Medium	Low	Medium

One type of popular financial instrument that we don't include in this table is the mutual fund. Where do mutual funds fit into the list of investments? They are simply a type of investment that includes one or more of the investments described in the above table. Since mutual funds are made up of any or all of the investments shown in the table, they carry with them the underlying characteristics of those investments. For example, a mutual fund that invested in term deposits and GICs would carry the inherent income, growth, and risk characteristics of those investments.

The table above is a general guideline and does not represent hard-and-fast rules. For example, you can have a GIC investment that has high risk if it is obtained from a financial organization that is not insured by the Canada Deposit Insurance Corporation (CDIC) or by one of the various other organizations that provide insurance coverage of such investments. Even in Canada, in the past we have seen circumstances in which people thought a particular type of investment was low risk and was insured, only to discover that it was not. Just ask anyone who invested in GICs at the Principal Group of companies in Alberta in the 1980s. This was a large, supposedly stable group of investment companies. However, to the chagrin of many investors, their investments were found to be worthless when that financial organization collapsed amid reports of potential fraud, mismanagement, and other shenanigans.

It is always in your best interest to find out if your investment is insured and by whom. This should be one of the things you consider before you decide to make an investment.

Savings Accounts and Canada Savings Bonds

The safest and most straightforward investment that you can make is to place your money in a simple bank account or in a Canada Savings Bond (CSB).

Keep in mind that many "branchless banks" that are setting up shop in Canada, such as mbanx and Ing Bank, offer higher interest rates on savings accounts than most other financial institutions. Even so, in these days of low interest rates and low inflation, the returns on savings accounts are minimal.

You can purchase CSBs at most banks, earn interest income on them, and cash them in at any time. It is almost like having your money in a savings account that pays a better rate of interest.

There is not much more to discuss in terms of analysis or education when it comes to a savings account or a Canada Savings Bond.

There is relatively little risk with such an investment, since most bank accounts are insured by the Canada Deposit Insurance Corporation for up to $60,000, and the federal government guarantees the value of the Canada Savings Bond. Since there is little risk, the income earned is rather low. Given the current low rate of inflation in Canada, you can expect an interest rate of less than 2% on a savings account and with CSBs, rates of 3.75% for the 1998 series of bonds.

The growth potential? None, since there is no other increase in the value of the investment other than the interest that you will earn.

GICs and Term Deposits

The next types of investment are GICs (guaranteed investment certificates) and term deposits.

These are usually offered by banks, credit unions, and trust companies. You invest your money (usually a minimum amount, $500 to $1,000) in a term deposit (also known as a certificate of deposit) or a GIC for a fixed period of time, ranging from 30 days to five years or more.

You are paid a guaranteed rate of interest on your investment at the end of the investment period on a term deposit, and on a monthly, quarterly, or yearly basis on a GIC.

Buying nonredeemable GICs or term deposits means you cannot cash them in during the fixed term. Redeemable GICs or term deposits can be redeemed during their term, although there is sometimes a penalty. You generally get a lower rate of interest on the latter type of investment.

GICs and term deposits are attractive alternatives to savings accounts and CSBs, since they often offer a higher rate of interest. The risk is low if the GIC or term deposit is taken out in Canadian dollars and has a term of less than five years, since it will likely be insured by the CDIC or similar deposit insurance corporation. The CDIC does not insure term deposits if the investment period is longer than five years.

Stocks

If your objectives and risk profile suggest that you would like to enhance your opportunity for growth, you might want to think about investing in the stock market.

Stocks are the primary means by which you can "grow your money." In the long term prior to the market downturn in 1998, the stock market in Canada, the United States, and elsewhere was roaring, with the result that some people saw average increases in the overall value of their stock investment of 20% to 30% or more. With the decrease in stock prices in 1998, many investments lost value. However, most investment advisors believe that in the long term, regardless of short-term fluctuations, the overall trend is for equities to rise.

Yet by the same token, any particular stock investment can turn out to be disastrous when the price falls. Just ask anyone who still held shares in Bre-X when it collapsed, or in the Ottawa-based telecommunications company Gandalf when it went out of business in 1997.

You can invest in either common or preferred shares,

in which case your return comes from any dividend declared on the shares as well as any increase (or decrease) in the stock's value on a stock exchange. Common shares normally give you voting rights within the organization, while preferred shares do not. But this is probably a moot point, since your vote will have little influence on what the company does.

So what is the difference between common and preferred shares? Typically, the value of a common stock will fluctuate more on the stock market compared to a preferred stock, thus providing greater opportunity for growth or more of a risk of a loss. Preferred shares offer a stated dividend, making them a good investment for a regular stream of income when compared to common stocks.

There are various terms used to describe particular "categories" of stocks based on the risk, income, and growth profile of the investment. Although there is no definitive list, here are some of the categories you are likely to hear about:

- **Blue chip stocks**
  A term used to describe large, solid, stable, and reliable companies whose stock price is not expected to fluctuate much over time. Examples are Bell Canada and General Motors. Such stocks usually offer regular income in the form of dividends, low risk due to the stability of the company, and regular growth in the value of the stock due to a steady stream of growth in the underlying value of the company.

- **Large cap stocks**
  Large cap stocks are stocks that aren't considered to be blue chip because they don't have a consistent history of dividend income and might be a bit more risky—but that have a market value of billions of dollars. There is a ready market in various stock exchanges for such stocks, making them fairly low-risk, reliable investments.

- **Small caps**
  The term "small caps" is used to describe the stock of small, startup companies or large-scale new ventures. Such stocks might or might not be traded on major stock exchanges. The risk is higher, but they offer more opportunity for growth in the stock value. The income

stream from dividends is usually nonexistent or inconsistent.

- **Emerging growth stocks**
  Emerging growth stocks are stocks that have a good chance of growing faster than the stock market in general. Often found in hi-tech computer or biotechnology sectors.

- **Speculative stocks**
  Stocks that are rather risky are called speculative.

Bonds

Bonds are investments in the debt of a company or government body. You derive a regular stream of interest income on the debt, as well as on any fluctuation in the market value of the debt instrument itself, should you sell it prior to maturity.

In essence, a company or government issues a bond to borrow money—and they promise to pay regular interest on the bond, as well as pay off the amount owing on the bond after a fixed period of time.

Bonds issued by the Canadian government, most provincial governments, or the municipal government are very low risk, whereas bonds issued by corporations will often match the risk profile of the stock of those companies.

Mutual Funds

As we mentioned earlier, mutual funds are just a combination of various investments. We discuss mutual fund concepts in appendix C.

Other Financial Investments

Of course, the investments we've described on the last few pages are only a sample of what's available. Venture into the world of finance, and you can discover many other financial investments, ranging from commodities to gold bars to futures contracts. Clearly, the scope of these other investments is beyond this book.

That isn't to say that these other alternatives aren't available to you—they are. And certainly you can use the Internet to learn about other types of investments. If you do, keep in mind the key caveat of investing: for any investment, assess its income, growth, and risk characteristics in light of your own financial objectives and investor profile.

The Role of the Internet in Investing

The Internet can help you choose which investments you should be considering, but you shouldn't become overly reliant on the technology.

Your personal judgment and analysis of potential investments are key to deciding what best suits your particular financial situation and investment objectives.

Having said that, there are a number of organizations that provide online information and interactive tools to help you determine the types of investments that are best for you. These tools will teach you about some of the financial implications and risk factors we mentioned in this appendix and how these factors should guide your investment decisions.

When it comes to your investments, the Internet can help you in several ways:

- **learning** more about investing
- **deciding** what to invest in
- **buying and selling** the investments you are interested in
- **monitoring** the value of your RRSP and/or other investments.

APPENDIX C

Mutual Fund Concepts

HIGHLIGHTS

- A mutual fund is a pooled investment that carries certain growth, income, and risk characteristics.

- In order to assess whether a mutual fund fits your investment objectives, you need to examine the types of investments that make up the fund as well as its associated growth, income, and risk profile.

- Common types of mutual funds include equity funds, bond/income funds, money market funds, mortgage funds, dividend funds, resource funds, specialty funds, and balanced funds.

- Mutual funds are attractive to Canadians for several reasons, including their flexible risk, low cost, and the management talent that oversees the performance of the fund.

- When evaluating a mutual fund, consider the fund's portfolio and its risk factor, its management fees and commissions, the reputation of the organization where you are purchasing the fund, and the reputation of the fund management team.

Many Canadians who choose not to invest directly in the stock or bond market, and who wish to invest in something other than CSBs, GICs, or term deposits, have turned to mutual funds instead, fuelling what has become an explosive industry.

Of course, many invest in mutual funds without having an understanding of exactly what these investments are.

Mutual Fund Basics

If, like many Canadians, you plan to invest your money in mutual funds, you should have a good understanding of what mutual funds are, and of the risk, income, and growth characteristics of the various funds available to you.

Mutual funds are, quite simply, "pooled investments." Rather than buying your own stocks, bonds, or even gold, you and many other people buy into a fund that is managed by a professional investor. The investor places this pool of money into investments that match the particular objective of the fund. You trust the good judgment and reputation of this investor to make investments that give a good return for your money.

It's as if you and a bunch of friends got together, pooled your money, and decided to use the funds to buy a few stocks, bonds, GICs, or bars of gold. You then hire a buddy who has some great experience in the investment world to oversee your investments and to continually assess whether they should be shifted to something else.

There are over 1,800 mutual funds available in Canada. Every mutual fund has a specific objective with respect to risk, income, and growth, all of which are detailed in a formal "prospectus," a document that summarizes everything about the fund. Your task as an individual investor is to ensure that you invest in mutual funds that match your own investment objectives.

But even before covering those topics, it is probably useful for you to understand the Canadian mutual fund industry.

Canadian Mutual Fund Companies

There are several distinct types of mutual fund companies in Canada. They include:

- **Subsidiaries of large banks and trust companies**
  All of the big banks and trust companies in Canada sell their own mutual funds directly to their customers. You can purchase a mutual fund from them simply by walking into your local bank branch.

  However, it is important to recognize that you are not dealing directly with the banks, but with special mutual fund investment companies that they have set up. This is an important point, for it directly impacts the type of protection on your investment. More about that later.

  You should read the fine print when dealing with one of these companies. For example, at their Web site you can read about the mutual funds offered by the Royal Bank of Canada. But it is only by reading the fine print that you are told that "Royal Mutual Funds are sold by Royal Mutual Funds Inc., a member of Royal Bank Financial Group...." Similarly, visit the Canada Trust Web site, and you will discover in the fine print that "The funds are distributed by CT Investment Management Group Inc., a subsidiary of Canada Trust...."

- **Mutual fund companies**
  There are other companies not affiliated or owned by major banks and trust companies, but which are independent firms or subsidiaries of other Canadian or U.S. financial organizations.

  Names you will encounter include Mackenzie Financial, Trimark, Altamira, AGF, Talvest, and many others. These are companies solely in the business of establishing mutual funds and offering these funds for sale to the public.

- **Insurance companies**
  Some insurance companies offer mutual funds directly for sale through subsidiaries, similar to what banks and trust companies have done. Others offer a special form of mutual fund called "segregated funds," which are often sold by their life insurance agents. These mutual funds differ from other mutual funds in that they have a "guarantee clause" that limits your risk. You can buy segregated funds directly, but some are tied to life insurance policies or retirement plans.

Where Can You Buy Mutual Funds?

This might seem like a silly question, but it isn't. There are some very real distinctions in terms of where you can go to buy particular mutual funds.

If you are interested in a particular fund, one of the first things you must do is determine whether you can purchase it directly from the fund company or whether you must go through some third party, such as a financial planner, broker, or agent.

Let's put things into perspective:

- Banks and trust companies sell their mutual funds directly through their bank branches, through 1-800 numbers, and online.

- Many mutual fund companies will sell their funds only through the agents, independent financial planners, and brokers who represent them. Companies that fall into this category are AGF and Trimark.

- Other mutual fund companies, such as Altamira, Caldwell, Phillips, Hager & North, Saxon Funds, Sceptre Mutual Funds, and Scudder Funds of Canada, sell their funds directly through 1-800 numbers, in addition to selling them through agents, financial planners, and brokers. They have become known as discount fund companies.

- Finally, there are a few fund companies, such as Investors Group, that sell their funds only through their own direct-sales representatives.

Do You Need Financial Advice?

Why is there a difference in the way that funds are sold? Why can you purchase some directly and not others? Why should you have to deal with a financial planner or broker to purchase some funds and not others? Does this impact on the quality of the investment?

The answers to these questions have to do with the way the mutual fund industry has evolved.

Originally, most, if not all, mutual funds were sold directly through brokers, financial planners, or agents of the companies that established the funds. The role of these people was to ensure that the investor had adequate information to assist them in selecting funds appropriate to their financial objectives. To fund this "middleman," a commission (referred to as a "load") was charged on the sale of the fund.

This structure began to change with the arrival of discount fund companies—organizations that sold their funds directly through their own representatives, often through a local office or with a 1-800 number. By doing so, they often eliminated the commission paid to the financial advisers. Thus the "no-load" fund was born.

This distinction is still evident today—you can choose to use the financial advice offered by particular fund companies if you are interested in their product, or you can choose to go the no-load route.

But you should also note that the emergence of the Internet in the world of finance is blurring this distinction even further. One example is E*Trade Canada, a company that offers online stock trading and mutual fund sales directly through the Internet. At their Web site you can purchase mutual funds from AGF, an organization that has historically only sold its funds through financial planners and brokers.

What Does a Mutual Fund Company Do?

The best way to understand this question is to consider what happens when a new mutual fund is created.

In 1997 Altamira announced two new funds, the Altamira T-Bill Fund and the Altamira Short Term Canadian Income Fund. Let's look at the former.

When creating the T-Bill Fund, Altamira established several objectives for the fund. As they note in the description of the fund on their Web site, the fund would be for "conservative investors who can sustain only minimum risk" and who might need "emergency cash reserves" or who are "saving for short-term goals."

In effect, the specified fund objective is to minimize the risk of any loss in the value of the investment, provide the ability for investors to obtain their money from the fund as quickly as possible should they need it, while providing more income on the investment than if investors had placed their money in a savings account or other type of cash investment.

The specific investment strategy established was for the fund to "invest exclusively in Government of Canada Treasury Bills or other short-term debt instruments of, or guaranteed as to the principal and interest by, Canadian federal or provincial governments denominated in Canadian dollars."

A professional investor named Frances Connelly, a vice president at Altamira, was assigned as the fund manager. With eighteen years of investment experience, five of those years at Altamira, she also manages the Altamira Short Term Government Bond Fund as well as having managed the Altamira Dividend Fund.

What did she invest the money in? A look at the Web site for the fund disclosed that it held a mix of Canadian government treasury bills (a form of government bond), which offered various levels of interest.

What is her role? To oversee the strategy of the fund and manage its activities, in order to achieve the stated goals of the fund. And, if you invest in the fund, you are deciding that you will place your faith in her ability to do that.

What does the mutual fund company Altamira do? In effect, it establishes and then manages many mutual funds in addition to this T-Bill fund, each of which has a manager that oversees that fund. The manager of each fund, together with his or her investment team, oversees the fund on a day-to-day basis, deciding what new investments to purchase for the fund to improve its performance and selling or "divesting" other investments that are performing poorly.

What Mutual Funds Invest In

Most mutual funds are established in order to fit a particular investment profile and have specific objectives. In effect, your money is placed in investments that have particular growth, income, and risk characteristics that match the objectives of the fund as much as possible.

Clearly, any mutual fund bears the very characteristics of the investments it holds. The Altamira T-Bill fund described above would be very low risk, given its investments in T-Bills, but would offer little in the way of growth potential, since such investments don't grow in value over time.

When trying to determine what type of mutual fund to

purchase, you should examine the type of assets that make up the fund you are considering. For example, does it invest in common stock, debt, or mortgages? Other types of investments? What are the characteristics of those investments, in terms of risk, growth, and income?

It isn't easy figuring out where to place your money, given that there are hundreds of mutual funds available for sale in Canada, each of which is based on a different mix of assets, promises a different rate of return, and has a different risk profile.

ND. are available for sale in Canada, each of which is based on a different mix of assets, promises a different rate of return, and has a different risk profile.

Nonetheless, you will discover that mutual funds can be grouped into several basic categories, as seen in the table on pages 218 and 219.

Within these categories you can find several sub-categories, based on whether the fund is based in Canadian, U.S., or international investments.

Net Asset Values

When you start to deal with mutual funds, you will have to become familiar with the term net asset value (NAV), which we mentioned in chapter 9. If you turn to the financial pages of various newspapers, you will discover that they often print the previous day's NAV for various mutual funds.

When you invest in a fund, you buy a certain number of units. If you invest $10,000 in a fund, and the current NAV is $2, you will own 5,000 units in the fund.

The NAV is the current value of one "unit" in a mutual fund, the value of which is based on its underlying assets. So if your mutual fund invests in gold, your NAV goes up and down as the price of gold rises and falls. If the mutual fund invests in a wide variety of stocks, the NAV will go up and down with the market value of those stocks.

The NAV can go up or down for two other reasons. First, income earned on the investments held in a mutual fund is often reinvested back into the mutual fund, rather than distributed to each mutual fund owner. This increases the NAV of the fund. Second, as we will see below, most mutual funds carry some type of management fee and are often charged other expenses that must be paid either by the income earned within the fund or by the sale of some assets, which decreases the NAV.

Type of fund	What it invests in...	Your return comes from...	Risk profile
Equity	Stocks of publicly traded or privately held companies.	Growth in the value of the stocks held plus any income from dividends declared on those stocks.	Medium to high, depending on type of stocks invested in.
Bond/Income	Bonds of publicly traded or privately held companies.	Primarily interest income on the bonds held plus any growth in the underlying value of the bond.	Low to medium, depending on the types of companies that have issued the bonds.
Money market	Government or corporate debt, that is, treasury bills or other forms of debt.	Interest paid on the debt plus any growth in the underlying value of the investment.	Low to medium. Most government-based money market funds are extremely low risk. The risk can be a bit higher if invested in commercial paper offered by the corporate sector.
Mortgage	Commercial or residential mortgages.	Income earned on the mortgages in the form of interest paid on the mortgages plus any growth in the underlying value of the mortgages.	Medium to high, depending on the type of mortgage held and the types of companies involved. For example, a mortgage fund that holds mortgages on speculative commercial properties is more risky than one that holds straightforward personal real estate mortgages.

Type of fund	What it invests in...	Your return comes from...	Risk profile
Dividend	Preferred or common shares of public or private companies that have a consistent dividend payment record.	Income earned on dividends on these shares plus any growth of the underlying value of the shares.	Low to medium, depending on the type and background of the companies that make up the portfolio.
Resource	Gold, silver, or other resources.	Income primarily from fluctuations in market value of particular resources.	High.
Specialty	Investments in a particular sector, that is, resource stocks and bonds of a particular industry such as oil or gas.	Income from stocks, revenue from bonds/debt instruments, plus growth in underlying asset value.	Varies depending on industry and asset mix.
Balanced funds	A mix of stocks and bonds.	Income from stocks, revenue from bonds/debt instruments, plus growth in underlying asset value.	Varies.

What Makes Up the Income, Growth, and Risk Profile of a Mutual Fund?

Key to your selection of a particular mutual fund is determining whether it fits the income, growth, and risk characteristics that you seek in an investment. The type of underlying investment held in a fund—stocks, bonds, debt, etc.—will have a definite impact on the type of income, growth, and risk associated with the fund.

Consider three extremes: a mutual fund that invests in debt issued by the government of Canada, one that invests in precious metals such as gold, silver, and platinum, and one that invests in the shares of new, small Canadian companies.

Obviously, the value of the first fund will remain steady since the value of debt—say, a government bond—issued by the Government of Canada does not fluctuate greatly. Such a fund would offer a steady stream of income from the interest payments on the debt, very low risk, and little prospect for growth and would be chosen by someone who simply wants a secure investment that promises a steady stream of income.

The value of the precious metals mutual fund will fluctuate according to the market values of these precious metals. It would offer good potential for growth, should the value of precious metals increase on worldwide markets—yet would obviously carry a fair degree of risk, due to the large fluctuations that can occur in the metals markets. The potential for regular income is very small, since the only income that would be derived on the fund would be from an increase in the market value of the precious metals in the fund.

Finally, a mutual fund that invested in the stocks of small Canadian startup companies would have high risk, due to the potential for significant fluctuations in the stock price of those companies. It would likely offer a low level of regular income since such companies would not be regularly distributing and declaring dividends. Yet the opportunity for growth in the value of the fund is high, since the inherent value of the fund is directly linked to the potential of these small companies to grow larger over time.

Clearly, the assessment of the income, growth, and risk characteristics of any particular mutual fund is dependent upon the underlying investments that make up that fund.

Are Mutual Funds Insured?

Investments in mutual funds are *not* insured in the same way that bank deposits are. This means that if a mutual fund company fails, you could lose all or some of the value of your investment.

This is true regardless of where you bought the fund. Many people mistakenly believe that mutual funds they purchase from a bank are safer than those from a mutual fund company—in the belief that the regular deposit insurance at their bank applies to their mutual funds.

But this is not true. As we noted previously, even if you are buying a mutual fund *at* a bank, it doesn't mean you've bought it *from* a bank. Once again, read the fine print at the bank or trust company Web site—you will note that you've bought the fund from a subsidiary of the bank, and that it is not insured. For example, consider what is posted at the Royal Bank of Canada and Canada Trust Web sites, respectively:

> Royal Mutual Funds are available only to residents of Canada. Royal Mutual Funds are sold by Royal Mutual Funds Inc., a member of Royal Bank Financial Group, and are not insured by the Canada Deposit Insurance Corporation, the Régie de l'assurance dépôts du Québec or any other deposit insurer nor guaranteed by Royal Bank or Royal Trust.

> The Funds are distributed by CT Investment Management Group Inc. ("CT IMG"), a subsidiary of Canada Trust, and are not insured by the Canada Deposit Insurance Corporation, The Régie d'assurance-dépôt du Québec, or any other government deposit insurer, or guaranteed by Canada Trust.

Mutual funds certainly carry a higher risk profile than bank deposits, GICs, term deposits, and other monetary investments that are directly insured, even if the assets that exist in a mutual fund consist of those particular types of investments.

What is the nature of the risk? The risk is twofold:

- Each mutual fund invests in certain things—stocks, bonds, precious metals, etc. You have a risk in the decrease of the value of your investment in the fund, should the value of the investments held in the fund decrease.

- Second, there is the potential risk, however small, of the failure of the mutual fund company.

There is not much you can do with the first type of risk, other than to carefully think through the risk characteristics of a particular mutual fund that you might be interested in.

For the second type of issue, you should be aware that the Canadian Investor Protection Fund (CIPF) might apply to your fund—always check!

The CIPF is managed by the Canadian investment industry and provides coverage for individuals making investments through members of the CIPF. The CIPF covers customers' losses of securities and cash balances, including mutual funds, up to $500,000. However, the amount of cash losses that you can claim as part of the $500,000 limit may not exceed $60,000. Visit their Web site for more detailed information.

Note that coverage only applies if a particular institution becomes insolvent. Once again, we must stress that coverage doesn't apply to the normal fluctuations in the value of your fund. If you invest in a fund that invests in stocks, and the stock market crashes, the value of your mutual fund goes down accordingly. You aren't covered for this risk.

Sometimes, when a mutual fund company fails, other mutual fund companies step in to take over the assets of the fund—resulting in little risk to the holder of those funds. Fortunately, it is rare for a mutual fund company to fail.

Remember the importance of not only diversifying your money by investing in different types of investments, but also of diversifying when it comes to different companies: spread them out to get maximum insurance coverage.

APPENDIX C: Mutual Fund Concepts

The Pros and Cons of Mutual Funds

Clearly, there must be some benefit to mutual funds or there would not have been such an explosion in their growth across Canada and around the world. What do you gain by investing in mutual funds? Several things:

Management Talent

Once you have decided which mutual funds you want to invest in, you are, in effect, relying on the decisions made by investment professionals. It is their full-time job to make the right choices in managing the investments in the fund—they continually decide what investments should be bought and sold by the fund in their efforts to meet the objectives of the fund.

Flexible Risk

There are all kinds of different mutual funds to match different risk objectives. In Canada, there are in excess of 1,800 mutual funds that you can choose from. This means that you can pick and choose the types of mutual funds that best match your particular risk factors, and diversify your portfolio so that it carries both low-risk and high-risk funds, or a mixture of low-growth and high-growth funds.

Low Cost

One reason for the explosive growth of mutual funds is that they permit more Canadians, who might not otherwise be able to invest in anything much more sophisticated than bank term deposits, to invest in any number of different funds for a relatively low entry cost. You can invest in some mutual funds with investments starting as low as $500 or less, allowing you to diversify your investments beyond savings accounts or Canada Savings Bonds.

Yet, in spite of all the positive aspects of mutual funds, there are also some potential downsides.

We should repeat that when you invest in mutual funds, you are relying on the decisions made by an investment professional. You certainly hope that these people are good at what they do. But remember that professional investors make mistakes just like amateurs do. The fact that they are professionals does not mean they are perfect.

Here in Canada, we have seen some of the highest profile and most successful mutual fund managers fall from grace, as the performance of their particular fund goes from fabulous to terrible in the space of just a few years.

You should also be aware that, in one way or another, you are going to have to pay for the services of those investment professionals! You can end up paying in several ways:

- Management fees are deducted from the fund assets. Since your return comes from the growth in the value of the fund and also depends on the income it earns, the management fee, in essence, comes out of the value of your investment. Management fees range from $1/2$% to $2^1/_2$% or more and are charged on an annual or monthly basis against the total assets of the fund.

- "Front-end load" funds charge a commission on the sale when the person or firm sells you the fund. This means that some of your money goes to the salesperson rather than to your investment. This is in addition to the management fees charged annually to the fund.

- "Back-end load" funds assess a sales commission if you redeem (that is, sell) the fund within a certain time period, often within several years. So, while you might not pay a sales commission up-front, you still end up paying one when you want to get out of the fund! (You don't pay the commission if you hold on to the fund for the prescribed period of time.)

- Some fund firms charge other expenses related to the fund (such as printing, administration, and other fees) directly to the fund, while others take this money from the management fee that has been charged. You should always check a fund description when looking at the management fees, to see if other additional expenses are charged to the fund.

Before you invest in a particular fund, you should determine the type of fee and commission (load) that you might pay and compare this to other similar funds. Many newspaper reports, books, and certainly Web sites report on the management fees and other charges within a mutual fund.

APPENDIX C : Mutual Fund Concepts

Choosing a Mutual Fund

Look at a newspaper during mutual fund season, and you will see a mutual fund company boasting about its "historical rate of return," which is an indication of how well the fund has done in the past. If it shows a big number, many investors think it's a good investment and plunge ahead and purchase the fund.

You will often see a particular mutual fund company advertise these rates of return, often listing one-, three-, and five-year rates. This issue warrants special attention. "Historical returns" should not be the basis for an investment decision. If a fund has done well in the past, it does not mean that it will necessarily do well in the future. Past performance is not an indicator of the future performance of the fund, but it is not the only indicator. More important are the objectives of the fund and the types of assets in which it invests.

Assessing the Fund's Portfolio and Its Risk Factor

In appendix B we discussed how your decision to invest in CSBs, GICs, stocks, and/or bonds should depend on the appropriateness of each to your current financial situation and risk objectives.

Investing in mutual funds is no different. Purchasing a mutual fund that invests in government bonds is far less risky than one that buys a lot of gold stock out of penny mining companies! Therefore, you must learn to assess the underlying types of assets held in a particular mutual fund and determine if they match your desired risk profile.

Management Fees

You should also assess the fund's management fees. Are they low, high, or average compared to industry norms? Are you paying too much compared to other fund investments? A normal fee is considered by most to be about 2%.

Sales Commissions

Find out if there are front-end or back-end fees. If it is a no-load fund, are there other fees that might be charged that could reduce your investment? Also, make sure you examine back-end charges or penalties that might be placed on you should you seek to withdraw your money from the fund.

Reputation of the Organization

Consider the reputation and background of the organization as part of your evaluation of the fund.

Obviously, mutual funds from such financial institutions as banks and the larger mutual fund companies have more of a track record than some of the smaller, newer mutual fund companies on the block. But that's not to say that you are necessarily safer with a larger organization—keep in mind the comments we made earlier about the Canadian Investor Protection Fund.

Reputation of the Fund Management Team

Remember that once you have chosen a particular mutual fund, you are relying on someone else to make investment decisions for you. When analyzing different funds, it's important to factor in the reputation, background, and history of the fund management team—how well have they performed managing their funds and others they may have been involved in? Organizations that sell mutual funds usually include this information on their Internet sites.

Performance

Finally, after you have analyzed the fundamentals of the fund, you can return to the issue of performance. You might assume that if the fund has done well in the past, it might do well in the future, or conversely, that the past is no indication of what is to come. Whatever the case may be, past performance is one factor to consider when you weigh the future possibilities of any particular fund.

What It Comes Down To

When it comes right down to it, mutual funds can be a pretty good investment. There are a lot of individuals who are seeing some pretty good returns on their mutual fund investments.

Yet at the same time, there are others who aren't doing so well, simply because they have selected a mutual fund that is not performing well.

Mutual funds are not a panacea—they are like any other investment, in that some do well and others do not. The real key for you is to figure out which ones are appropriate for you and have a good likelihood of success.

Web Sites Mentioned in This Appendix

AGF Group of Funds	www.agf.ca
Altamira Investment Services	www.altamira.com
Canada Trust	www.canadatrust.com
Canadian Investor Protection Fund	www.cipf.ca
E*Trade Canada	www.canada.etrade.com
Investors Group	www.investorsgroup.com
Mackenzie Financial	www.mackenziefinancial.com
Phillips, Hager & North	www.phn.ca
Royal Bank of Canada	www.royalbank.com
Saxon Funds	home.inforamp.net/~saxon/index.html
Scudder Funds of Canada	www.scudder.ca
Talvest Mutual Funds	www.talvest.com
Trimark Mutual Funds	www.trimark.com

APPENDIX D

Learning About Investments on the Internet

HIGHLIGHTS

- You can use the Internet to understand more about cash-based and cash-equivalent offerings from various financial institutions.

- The Internet is an extremely useful place to learn about the fundamentals of mutual funds. In order to take full advantage of its potential, you will need to distinguish between those sites that want to educate you and those sites that simply want to sell you something.

- The Internet makes it possible for investors to access a wide range of information about the stock and bond markets. The sheer volume of information can often be overwhelming.

In this appendix we give you a short but concise outline of how you can use the Internet to better understand the world of financial investments.

Learning About Cash-Based Investments Online

As you put together your investment strategy, you will find that most financial experts recommend that you diversify your RRSP portfolio or ensure that your other investments are well diversified. This means that some portion of your overall savings should be in cash-based or cash-equivalent investments. You should therefore understand the options that exist for these investments and learn how to determine the income and risk associated with them.

The first thing to keep in mind is that many financial institutions have two categories of cash-based investments: those that are only available through an RRSP and those that are not eligible to be held in an RRSP. When using the Web to research cash-based investments, look for RRSP/retirement sections on the Web sites of financial organizations. This will help you identify those cash-based investments that qualify for your RRSP.

Savings Accounts

Most banks, credit unions, and trust companies provide online details about the types of savings accounts that they offer and the current rates.

For example, Scotiabank offers a useful section on their Web site that includes descriptions of their deposit accounts as well as the current rates:

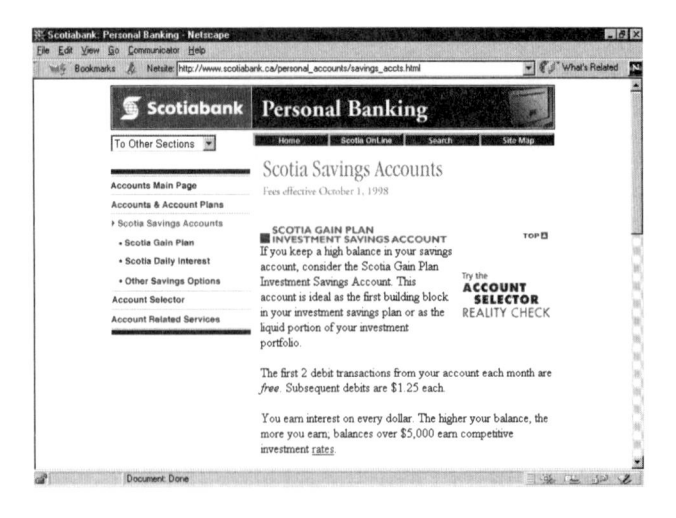

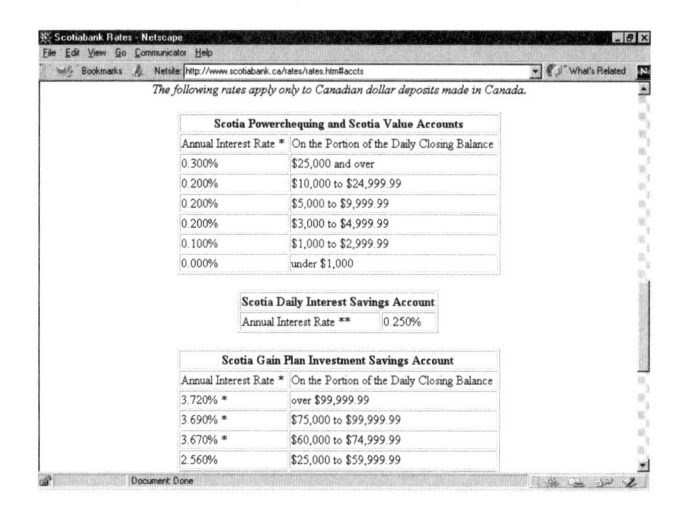

APPENDIX D: Learning About Investments on the Internet

The following rates apply only to Canadian dollar deposits made in Canada.

Scotia Powerchequing and Scotia Value Accounts

Annual Interest Rate *	On the Portion of the Daily Closing Balance
0.300%	$25,000 and over
0.200%	$10,000 to $24,999.99
0.200%	$5,000 to $9,999.99
0.200%	$3,000 to $4,999.99
0.100%	$1,000 to $2,999.99
0.000%	under $1,000

Scotia Daily Interest Savings Account

Annual Interest Rate **	0.250%

Scotia Gain Plan Investment Savings Account

Annual Interest Rate *	On the Portion of the Daily Closing Balance
3.720% *	over $99,999.99
3.690% *	$75,000 to $99,999.99
3.670% *	$60,000 to $74,999.99
2.560%	$25,000 to $59,999.99

If you are going to place some of your money into such an account, then find out whether the account is insured. Most banks and credit unions are insured through insurance corporations such as the Canada Deposit Insurance Corporation (CDIC) for banks and various provincial corporations for credit unions. If you are dealing with a smaller financial institution, however, be sure to find out if your deposits are covered by some type of insurance. Often this information is included on the organization's Web site, if one exists. This information should be factored into your overall assessment of the risk of your investment.

Canada Savings Bonds

You can learn a lot about Canada Savings Bonds at the federal government Web site for CSBs. This Web site gives the current rates for CSBs as well as a FAQ (frequently asked question summary) about using CSBs in your RRSP (see page 232).

1999 MUTUAL FUNDS AND RRSPs ONLINE

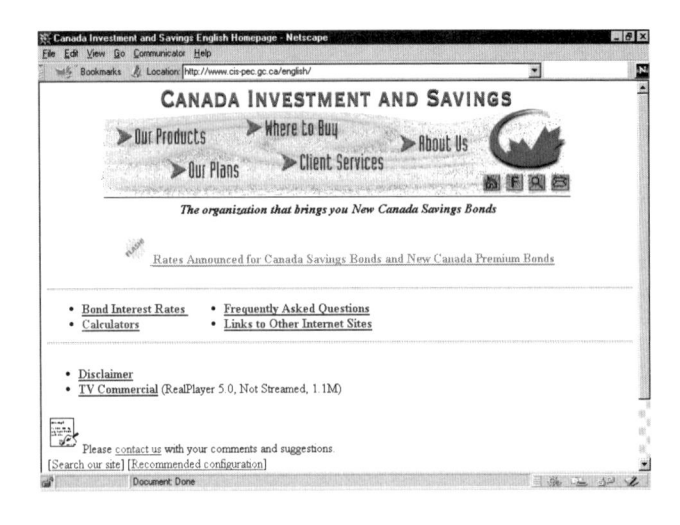

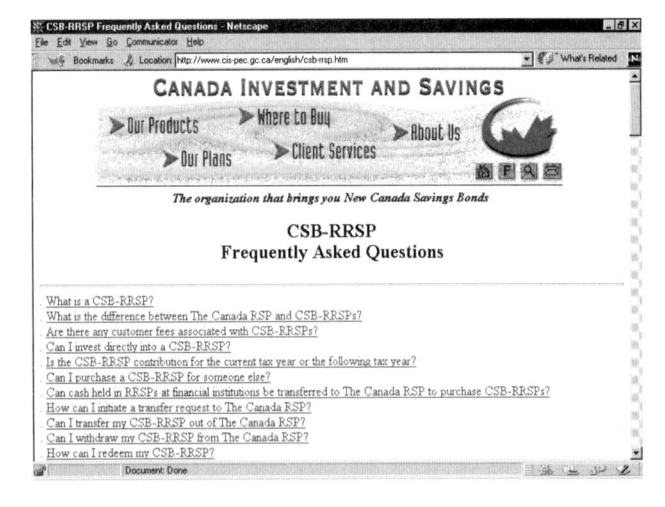

GICs/Term Deposits

If you are thinking of placing part of your RRSP investment in a GIC or term deposit, there are several things you should do. First, recognize that most bank, trust company, and credit union Web sites offer good descriptions of these particular investments, including any restrictions on withdrawal of the funds, RRSP eligibility, and other issues. For example, at the Web site for Vancouver City Savings Credit Union (VanCity), they have descriptions of their term deposits:

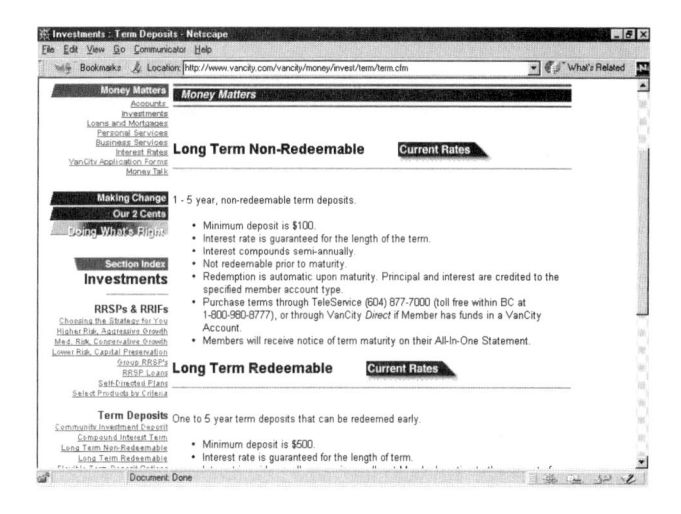

APPENDIX D: Learning About Investments on the Internet

You can also learn about their rates:

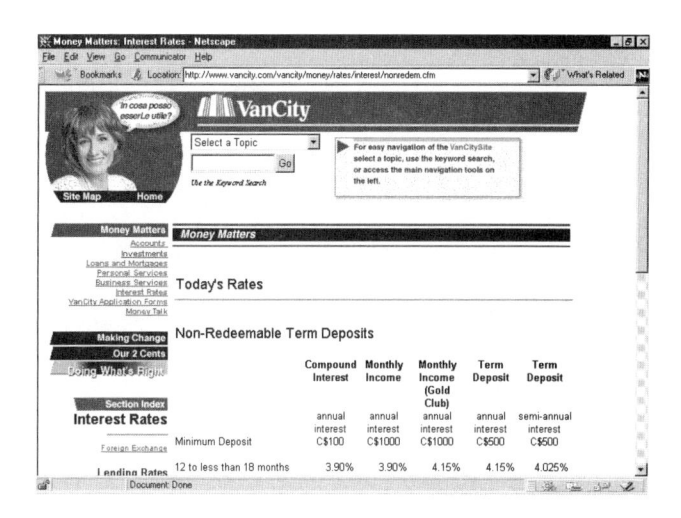

Learning About Mutual Funds Online

Survey after survey indicate that there is a pressing need for Canadians to know more about the basics of mutual funds. There is no doubt that many of us rush into such investments without really thinking about what we are doing.

It is important to take the time to understand the fundamentals of mutual funds before investing in them. If you want to learn more, you will discover that there is a lot of good educational material available online.

Many of the retirement sites we outlined in appendix A are good starting points, since they often provide basic background information on mutual funds and how they work. But as we pointed out, you have to learn to distinguish between the sites that are simply sales oriented and the ones that provide truly useful background and educational information.

As you tour the Internet to learn more about mutual funds, keep the following caveat in mind: your goal is to find the sites that provide good, concise information, not the sites that simply want to sell you something. We think that you will quickly develop the ability to know the difference between useful, nonbiased information and the down-and-dirty sales pitch. What should you look for? Focus on the Web sites that describe the fundamentals of mutual funds and that make it easy for you to find the answers to your questions.

Some of the more useful sites that fit this category are the following:

- The *Globe and Mail* GLOBEfund site features a comprehensive learning section, a glossary, a Getting Started section, an Online Investing section, and The Wise Investor section. The latter contains a variety of mutual fund articles by some of Canada's best-known financial authors, including Duff Young:

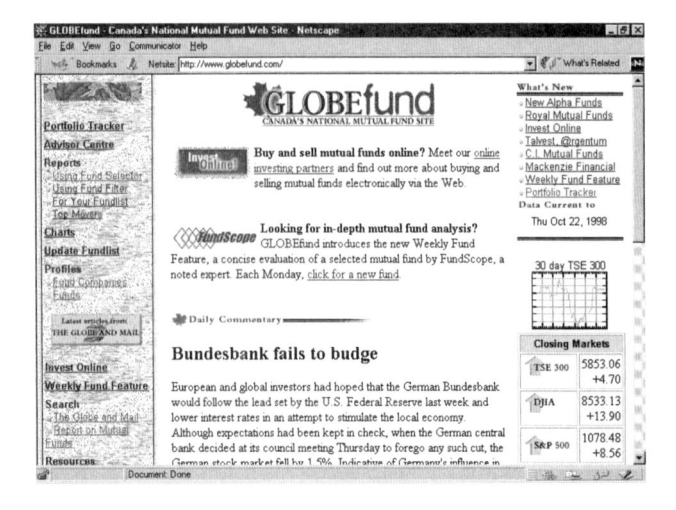

APPENDIX D: Learning About Investments on the Internet

- Several other Canadian newspaper sites include mutual funds sections. For example, The Money section on the CANOE Web site includes the article "Mutual Funds 101" by Jonathan Chevreau, a well-known writer for *The Financial Post*:

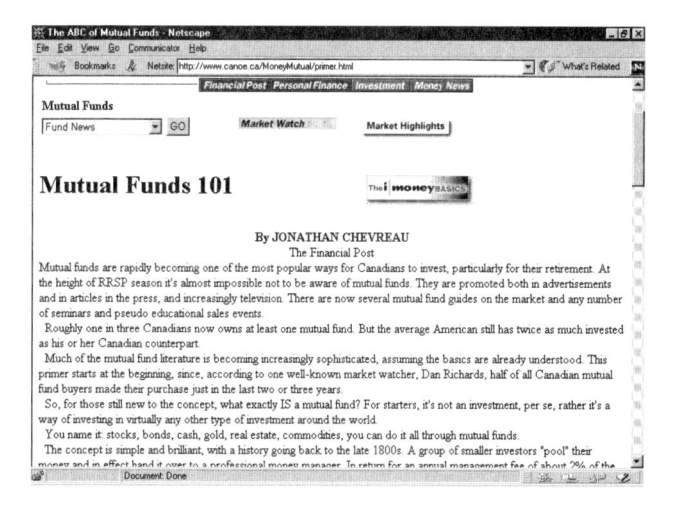

- Take a look at documents such as "Anatomy of a Mutual Fund?" and "10 Most Frequently Asked Questions About Mutual Funds" at the Investment Funds Institute of Canada site. The Institute represents the Canadian mutual funds industry. Its site also features an online glossary of mutual fund terms, which can be helpful when you encounter jargon you are not sure of.

- Check out "Invest Wisely: An Introduction to Mutual Funds" at the U.S. Securities and Exchange Commission Web site. Even though some of the specifics in that document are not appropriate for most Canadian investors, it is still a good introduction to the fundamentals of mutual funds.

- The Financial Concept Group, a Canadian Financial Planning organization, deserves plaudits for focusing less on the hard sell and more on education on its Web site. Its "Complete Guide to Mutual Funds" is a very good overview that is well worth a read:

1999 MUTUAL FUNDS AND RRSPs ONLINE

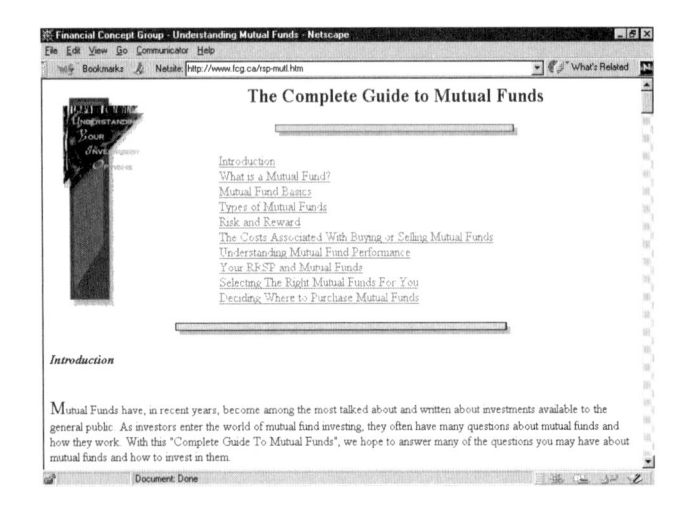

- Another good Canadian "financial supermarket" to visit is Sympatico's Personal Finance site, which includes a mixture of information sources and tools from iImoney as well as links to other investment sites, online discussion forums, advice from financial experts, and other information.

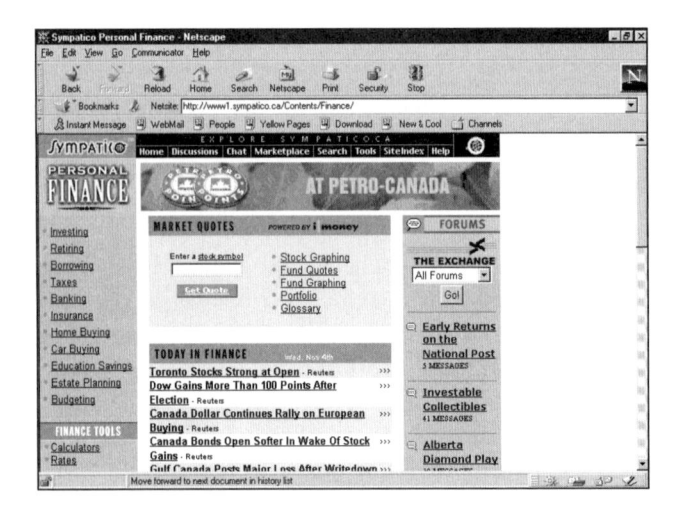

- Check out the Mutual Funds Switchboard, an excellent and comprehensive resource that lists various Canadian mutual fund information sites. It's one of the most comprehensive indexes available on the Web:

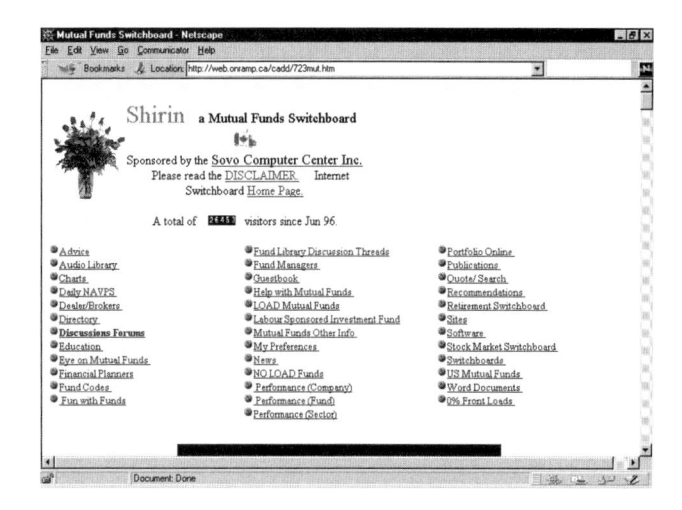

APPENDIX D: Learning About Investments on the Internet

- Spend some time in the Financial Pipeline. It includes some very useful educational material about mutual funds:

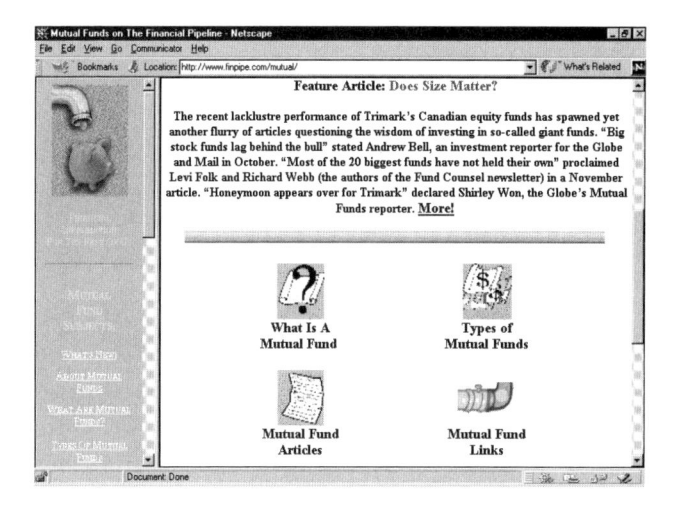

- Sometimes an Internet search can be very helpful. For example, simply typing "what is a mutual fund" into a popular Web search engine such as AltaVista Canada returns a lengthy list of useful sites to research.

Learning More About the Stock Market and Other Investments Online

It's easy to invest in a cash-based investment or mutual fund and earn a safe return, particularly if the mutual fund is cash based. But it's quite another to venture into the stock or bond market and expect solid, low-risk growth. There is a world of difference between the expertise required to invest in cash-based investments or mutual funds and that required to manage any kind of stock or bond investment. This is because the risk is higher in the stock market, and the complexity of what you become involved in can be much greater.

If you decide that you want to explore the world of the stock market and other financial investments, then your first task is to use the Internet to gain insight into some basic investment concepts. Fortunately, there is some good stuff out there.

The best places to start are the Web sites of independent organizations such as regulatory authorities and associations for individual investors.

The Investor Learning Centre of Canada has some excellent information that you can access on Canada Trust's CT Securities Web site. Featured on the site are investor "briefings" that describe how the stock, bond, and securities markets operate in Canada:

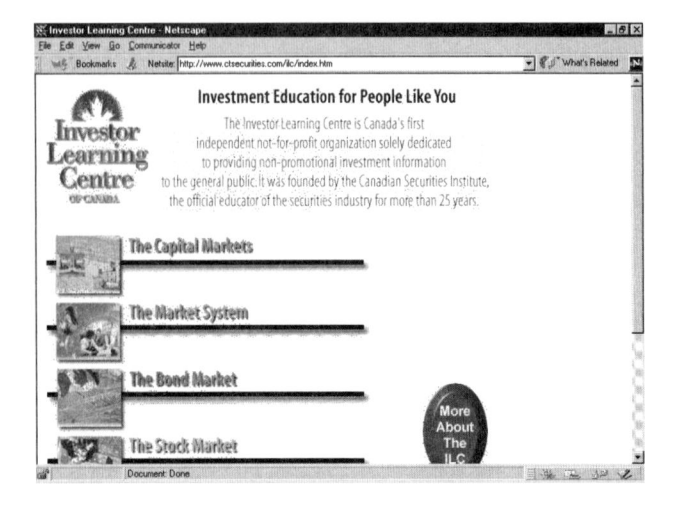

APPENDIX D: Learning About Investments on the Internet

Also check out the publication called "What Every Investor Should Know—A Handbook from the U.S. Securities and Exchange Commission" at the Securities and Exchange Commission (SEC) Web site. Look under the Consumer section. While written from a U.S. perspective, the document is a good introduction to the fundamentals of the stock market:

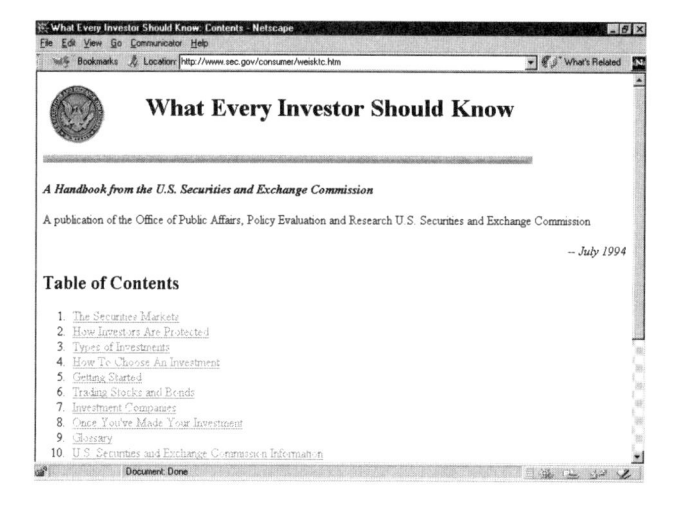

![Screenshot of "What Every Investor Should Know" webpage from the SEC, showing the title, subtitle "A Handbook from the U.S. Securities and Exchange Commission", publication information, date "July 1994", and a Table of Contents with 10 items: 1. The Securities Markets; 2. How Investors Are Protected; 3. Types of Investments; 4. How To Choose An Investment; 5. Getting Started; 6. Trading Stocks and Bonds; 7. Investment Companies; 8. Once You've Made Your Investment; 9. Glossary; 10. U.S. Securities and Exchange Commission Information.]

It offers pointers on how securities markets work, how to choose an investment, what is involved in trading stocks and bonds, and other related issues.

There are many other useful documents on the SEC Web site. For example, you should also take a look at "Invest Wisely: Advice from Your Securities Industry Regulators," which is a good overview of many things you should consider before plunging into the stock market.

You can learn how specific stock exchanges work by accessing their Web sites. The Vancouver Stock Exchange's Web site provides a good overview of its role, as do the Web sites belonging to the Montreal Stock Exchange and the Toronto Stock Exchange.

What about bonds? Check out Bonds Online. Although American, it does include "The Bond Professor," which can be a good source of information about the fundamentals of these investments:

239

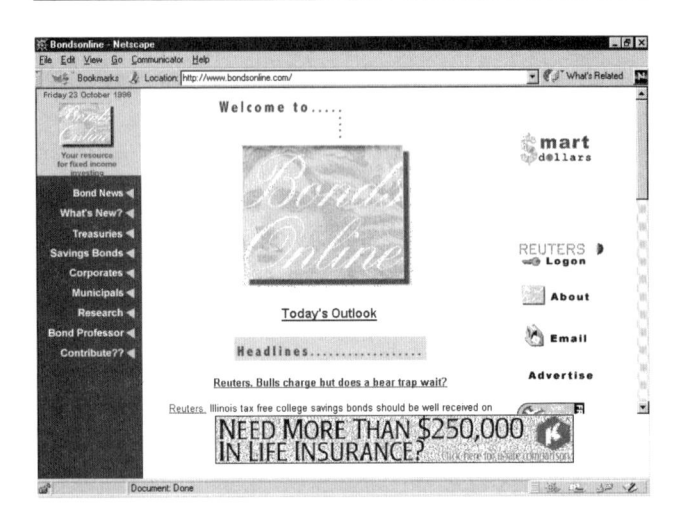

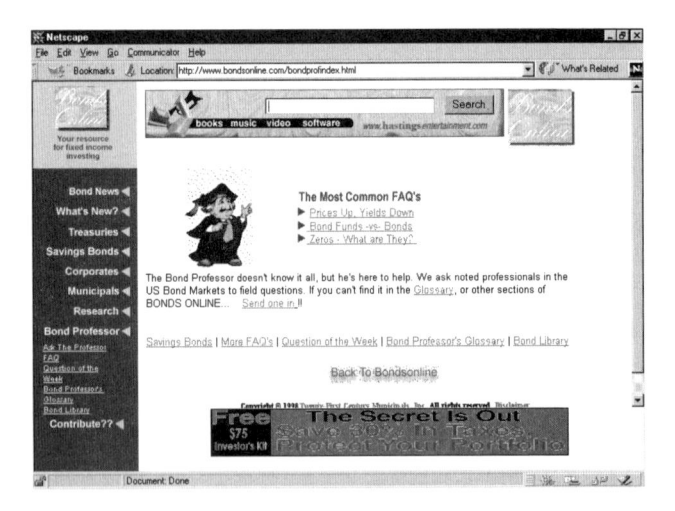

As for associations, check out the American Association of Independent Investors (AAII). Although the site has a U.S. focus, there is a lot of good investment information at both the basic and advanced levels. While some of the information is free, to get access to the full range of information available you must pay a fee:

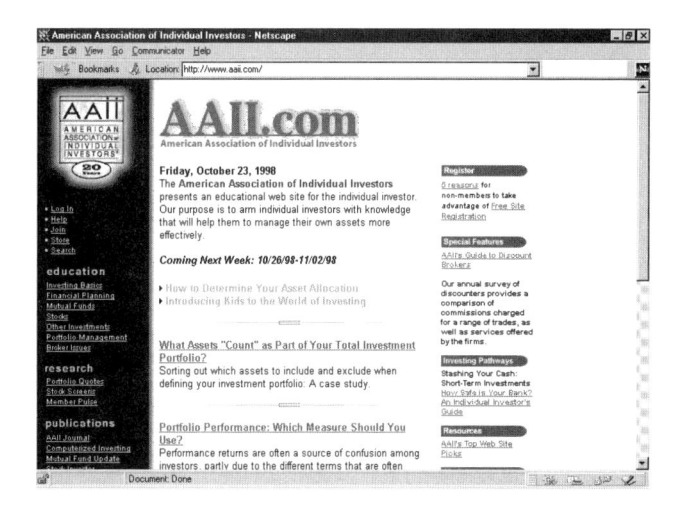

APPENDIX D : Learning About Investments on the Internet

There are many other similar associations online, but you need to be cautious. While there are associations like the AAII that have long track records, there are also the associations that are rather new or are scams and simply want your money.

The next document you should look at is the "Investment FAQ." Compiled on the Internet over a period of several years, it is a multipart document that deals with many different aspects of investments, including stocks, bonds, options, and other investments:

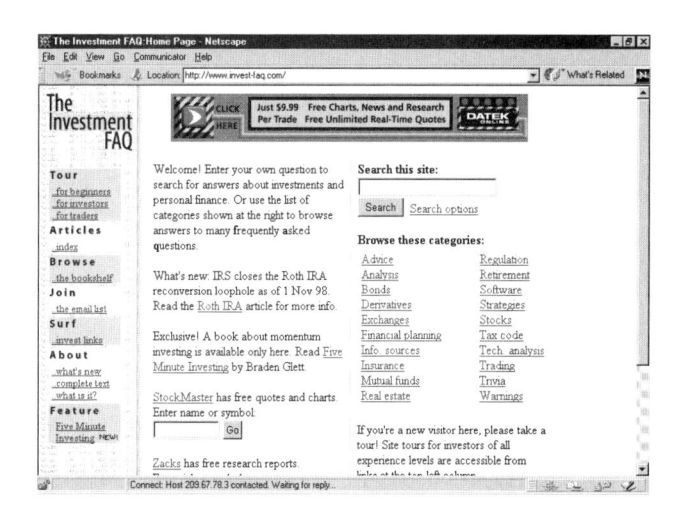

1999 MUTUAL FUNDS AND RRSPs ONLINE

This document provides additional background information to help you understand the stock market and other financial topics; there are also links to other sites. Specifically, consult the "Surf...invest links" section. That leads to a number of very comprehensive information sites where you can often find useful investor-education information:

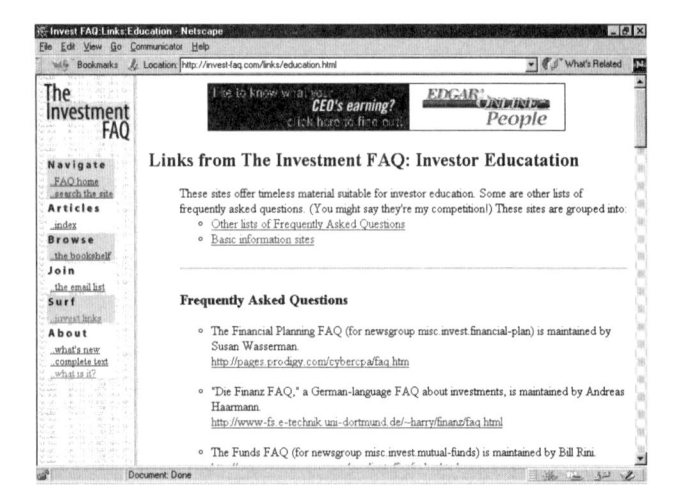

For example, from the FAQ we travelled to a site called "invest-o-rama," which features a fairly complex investor education area:

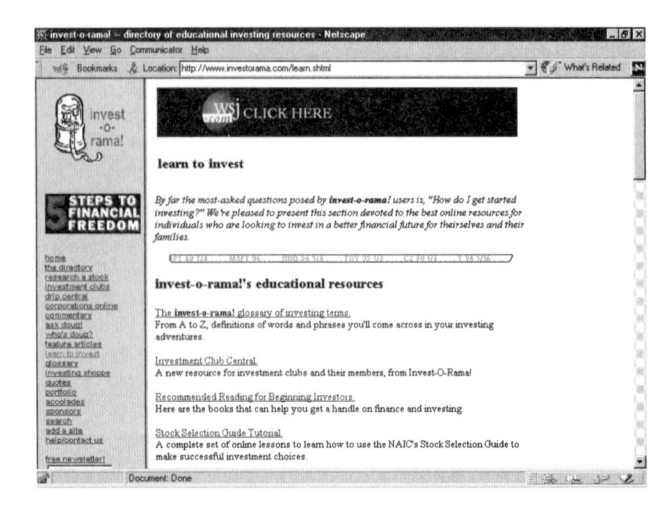

Conclusion

Using the Internet to learn about investing is a challenge in and of itself. The Investment FAQ notes that "the explosion in number of users and information providers on the Internet has yielded a mind-numbing quantity of sites with content related to personal finance and investments."

We couldn't have said it better.

Web Sites Mentioned in This Appendix

AltaVista Canada	www.altavistacanada.com
American Association of Individual Investors	www.aaii.com
Bonds Online	www.bondsonline.com
Canada Savings Bonds	www.cis-pec.gc.ca
Canada Deposit Insurance Corporation	www.cdic.ca
CANOE	www.canoe.ca
Financial Concept Group	www.fcg.ca
Financial Pipeline	www.finpipe.com
GLOBEfund	www.globefund.com
Investment FAQ	www.invest-faq.com
Investment Funds Institute of Canada	www.ific.ca
invest-o-rama	www.investorama.com
Investor Learning Centre of Canada	www.ctsecurities.com/ilc/index.htm
Montreal Stock Exchange	www.me.org
Mutual Funds Switchboard	web.onramp.ca/cadd/723mut.htm
Scotiabank	www.scotiabank.ca
Sympatico	www.sympatico.ca
Toronto Stock Exchange	www.tse.com
U.S. Securities & Exchange Commission	www.sec.gov
Vancouver City Savings Credit Union	www.vancity.com
Vancouver Stock Exchange	www.vse.ca

Index

AGF Group of Funds, 62, 70, 86, 139, 142, 143, 169, 213, 214, 215, 227
Alberta Securities Commission, 30
Alberta Stock Exchange (ASE), 29, 46
Alexander Personal Finance Search, 106, 108
All-Canadian Mutual Fund Guide, 189, 194
Altamira Investment Services, 62, 70, 85, 93, 136, 169, 213, 214, 215–216, 227
AltaVista, 61, 97, 105, 108, 237, 243
American Association of Independent Investors (AAII), 240–241, 243
American Express, 130, 131
Annuities, 191–193
Arthur Andersen, 189–190, 194
Asset allocation, *See* Asset mix
Asset mix, 42, 56–57
  and investment planning, 48–54
  and online questionnaires, 49–54
  utilizing online information, 45–48
Asset mix questionnaires, *See also* Online questionnaires, 41, 49–54
Asset mix tools,
  for mutual funds, 49–51
  general, 51–54
  limitations of, 54

Back-end load funds, *See also* Mutual funds, 224
Bank of Montreal, 113, 125, 131, 182
Bank of Nova Scotia, 86
Bell Canada, 207
Bell Charts, 89, 93
Bissett & Associates, 86
Blue chip stocks, *See also* Investment products and Stocks, 207
Bohr, Niels, 88
Bonds, *See also* Canada Savings Bonds, Investment products, 208
  and online research, *See also* Online research, Online investing, 95–107, 238–242
Bonds Online, 98, 108, 239, 243
Branchless banks, 205
Bre-X, 29, 206
British Columbia Securities Commission, 30, 38
Brokerages, full-service, 109
Business Wire, 104, 108
Buying/selling, on the Internet, *See* Online investing, Online trading services

Caldwell Investment Management, 214
Calgary Herald, 102
Canada Deposit Insurance Corporation (CDIC), 77, 80, 204, 205, 206, 231, 243
Canada Life, 52, 58
Canada NewsWire, 46, 104, 108
Canada Pension Plan (CPP), 177, 179, 180, 183, 185, 194
Canada Savings Bonds (CSBs), 205, 243

245

and online investing, *See also* Online investing, 137–138, 169
and online research, *See also* Online information, 231–232
Canada Stockwatch, 153, 169
Canada Trust, 50, 51, 58, 68, 70, 111, 113, 118, 131, 137, 153, 154, 169, 213, 221, 227
Canadian Bond Rating Service, 51
Canadian Corporate News, 46, 104, 108
Canadian Dealer Network, 46
Canadian Depository Securities, 106
Canadian Internet New User's Handbook, 6
Canadian Investors Protection Fund (CIPF), 113, 131, 222, 227
Canadian Magazine Publishers Association, 103, 108
Canadian Stock Market Reporter Inc., 153, 169
CANNEX, 71, 73, 80
CANOE (Canadian Online Explorer), 71, 75, 76, 80, 89, 93, 103, 104, 108, 127, 131, 139, 153, 154, 156, 169, 235, 243
Carlson On-line Services, 2, 46, 95, 98, 99, 108, 153, 157, 158, 169
Cash investments, on the Internet, 71–80
Cash-based investments, *See also* Investment products, Online investing, 202
and portfolio management, 134–138
on the Internet, 71–80
online research, 229–233
CBS MarketWatch, 98, 108
Charles Schwab, 25, 38, 111, 130, 132, 153, 169, 172
Chat sites, risks of, *See also* Online fraud, 21
CheckFree Quote Server, 153, 169
Chelekis, George, 19
Chevreau, Jonathan, 235
CIBC (Canadian Imperial Bank of Commerce), 73, 80, 125, 131
Citizens Bank of Canada, 52, 58
CNNfn, 98, 108, 129, 131

Commission calculators, *See also* Financial calculators, 116, 120–122
Commission-free mutual funds, *See also* Investment products, Mutual funds, 9
Commissions,
and online trading, 116–122
mutual fund, 118–120
Company research, on the Internet, 96–107
Comparator Systems, 15
Compound interest calculator, *See also* Financial calculators, 74
Computing Canada, 74
Con artists, *See* Scam artists, Online fraud
Conflict of interest, *See also* Online fraud, 19
Connelly, Frances, 216
Connor Clark & Lunn Investment Management, 86
Corporate Information, 98, 108
Credibility,
of online information, 25, 33–38
Credit Union Central Alberta, 79, 80
Credit Union Central of Canada, 79, 80
CT Investment Management Group, 213
CT Private Investment Counsel, 51
CT Securities, 118, 125, 132, 154, 169, 238
Cyber-schemes, *See* Online fraud

Daily Stocks, 95, 98, 101, 108
Debt-based investments, *See also* Investment products, Online investing, 203
Deloitte & Touche, 190, 194
Deposit insurance, *See also* Investment security, 77
Deposit Insurance Corporation of Ontario, 78, 80
Discount brokerages,
on the Internet, *See also* Commissions, Online trading services, 109, 110–111
Diversification, *See also* Asset mix, Investment concepts, 42, 48, 56–57, 200–201

INDEX

examples of, 44–45
Dynamic Mutual Funds, 63, 70

E*Trade, 112, 153, 169
E*Trade Canada, 9, 38, 55, 81, 83, 87, 89, 90, 93, 106, 109, 112, 115, 116, 117, 119, 121, 122, 124, 125, 132, 153, 159, 169, 215, 227
EDGAR (Electronic Data Gathering, Analysis and Retrieval System), 106, 108
Electric Library Canada, 104, 108
Electronic newsletters, risks of, *See also* Online fraud, 20
Emerging growth stocks, 208
Encarta Online Library, 105, 108
Equity-based investments, 203
Ernst & Young Canada, 65, 70, 190, 194
Excite, 97, 108
Exotic scams, *See also* Online fraud, 19–20

Fees, and online trading, *See also* Commissions, 116–122
FinanceWise, 106, 108
Financial advice, 214–215
Financial aggregators, 95, 98–102
Financial calculators, 59–69
  and the time value of money, 184
  risks of, *See also* Online fraud, 23
Financial Concept Group, 235, 243
Financial Pipeline, 51, 58, 237, 243
Financial Post, The, 102, 103, 127, 235
Financial planners, 55, 190
Financial search engines, 105–106
FIND/SVP, 112
First Canadian Mutual Funds, 60, 70, 182, 194
Forrester Research, 130, 131
Fortune, 103
Fraud, *See* Online fraud
Freerealtime.com, 153
Front-end load funds, *See also* Mutual funds, 224
Full-service brokerages, 109
Fundata Canada, 89, 93

The Fund Library, 34, 38, 81, 83, 86, 87, 91, 92, 93, 133, 139, 143, 145, 150, 169, 192–193, 94

Gambling, 172
Gandalf, 206
General Motors, 207
GIC calculators, *See also* Financial calculators, 134
GICs (Guaranteed Investment Certificates), *See also* Online investing, Investment products, 205–206
  market-linked, 75
  and online investing, 134
  and online research, 232–233
Globe and Mail, 34, 85, 128–129, 147, 188, 234
GLOBEfund, 34, 38, 47, 48, 58, 81, 83, 84, 85, 87, 90, 93, 127, 128–129, 132, 133, 139, 143, 147, 149, 169, 188, 194, 234, 243
Goldfarb Consultants, 3
Gomez Advisors, 130, 132
Good Health Online—A Wellness Guide For Every Canadian, 14
Government organizations, on the Internet, *See also* Online information, 106

Hepcoe Credit Union, 136, 169
Hongkong Bank of Canada, 111, 114, 126, 132
Hoover's Online, 98, 108
Human Resources Development Canada (HRDC), 179, 194
Hy-line Credit Union, 76, 80
Hypertechmedia, 74

i|money, 53, 58, 65, 73, 80, 139, 149, 169, 186, 189, 194
IE:Money, 189, 194
Inco, 99
Income taxes, and your RRSP, *See also* RRSPs, 65
Income-generating investments, 203
Industry Canada, *See also* Strategis, 99
Information security, 112
Information Service Dissemination Network, 46

Information skepticism, *See also* Online fraud, Online information, 15, 27–28
InfoSpace.com, 154, 169
Ing Bank, 205
Insider information, on the Internet, *See also* Online fraud, 30
Institute of Biological Engineering, 61
Insurance companies, and mutual funds, *See also* Mutual funds, 213
Integra Information, 98, 108
Interest rates, and the Internet, 72–73
Internet, *See also* Online information, Online investing
and company research, 96–107
and investment planning, 41–57
and misleading information, *See also* Online fraud, 23
and privacy, *See also* Online fraud, 23–24
and research, *See* Online investment research
and savings rates, 72–73
and securities regulators, 17, 28
and technical problems, 24–25
as an investment tool, 1–6
benefits of, 9–12
risks of, 12–33
benefits of, 7–12
its role in investing, 209
learning about investments, 229–243
risks of, 12–33
Internet fraud, *See* Online fraud
Internet security, *See also* Online information security, 112
Internet trading, *See* Online investing and Online trading services
InvesNET, 126, 132
Investext Research Bank, 98, 108
Investing, *See also* Online investing
and diversification, *See also* Diversification, 200–201
basic concepts of, 197–209
income, growth and risk, 199–200
kinds of investors, 198–202
the role of the Internet, 209
types of investment products, *See also* Online investing, 202–209
Investment advisors, 55, 190
unlicensed, *See also* Online fraud, 18–19
Investment Dealers Association of Canada (IDA), 32, 36
Investment education, 229–243
Investment FAQ, 243
Investment Funds Institute of Canada (IFIC), 83, 89, 93, 235, 243
Investment insurance, 113–114
Investment management, *See* Portfolio management
Investment mix, *See* Asset mix
Investment objectives, 41, 48–49, 55–56
Investment planning, *See also* Retirement planning and Online investment planning
and asset mix, 48–54, 56–57
and financial advice, 214–215
and Internet benefits, 9–12
and Internet risks, 12–33
theories of, 42–44
Investment product selection,
and asset mix, 56–57
and the Internet, 41–57
Investment products, 202–209
bonds, 208, 238–242
Canada Savings Bonds, 205, 231–232
cash-based, 202, 229–233
debt-based, 203
equity-based, 203
GICs (Guaranteed Investment Certificates), 205–206, 232–233
growth potential of, 203
income-generating, 203
mutual funds, 46–48, 208, 211–227, 233–237
other financial investments, 208–209
risk, 203–205
savings accounts, 205, 230–231
segregated funds, 213
stocks, 206–208, 238–242
term deposits, 205–206, 232–233
types of, 186

INDEX

Investment security, 76–79
Investment strategy, *See* Investment product selection
Investment tracking, *See* Portfolio management
INVESTools, 98, 102, 108
Investor Learning Centre of Canada, 238, 243
invest-o-rama, 98, 99–100, 108, 242, 243
Investors Group, 227

Janus Mutual Funds, 82
JournalismNet, 103, 108
Jupiter Communications, 112

KPMG Canada, 190, 194

Laidlaw Inc., 86
Large cap stocks, *See also* Investment products, Stocks, 207
Life income funds, *See also* Retirement planning, 176
Loaded mutual funds, *See also* Investment products, Mutual funds, 9, 84, 110, 118, 214–215
Lycos, 97, 108

Mackenzie Financial, 213, 227
Magna International Inc., 86
Management expense ratio (MER), *See also* Commissions, 84, 224, 225
Manitoba Senior Citizens Handbook, 179
Market Guide, 98, 108, 154, 169
Massachusetts Institute of Technology (MIT), 93
Mbanx, 205
Merrill Lynch, 172
Money, Inc., 103
Money.com, 154, 169
Montreal Stock Exchange, 36, 38, 46, 239, 243
Motley Fool, The, 29, 38
MSNBC, 123
Multex Investor Network, 98, 108
Munica, 134, 135, 169
Mutual fund asset classes, 82
Mutual fund companies, Canadian, 212–213
what they do, 215–216
Mutual Fund Switchboard, 83, 90, 92, 93, 236, 243

Mutual fund Web sites, what to look for, 84
Mutual fund(s), *See also* Investment products, 208
and daily net asset values (NAVs), 139, 217
and insurance companies, 213
and online analysis tools, *See also* Financial calculators, 47
and online asset mix tools, 49–51
and online discussion forums, 91–93
and online investing, *See also* Investment products, 81–93
and online portfolio management, 138–152
and online research, 46–48, 82–91, 233–237
and portfolio management software, 149–152
buying online, *See also* Online investing and Online trading, 124–125
categories of, 47, 218–219
choosing, 225–226
commissions, 118–120
concepts, 211–227
online comparison of, 83–88
online fund ranking, 43, 89
online performance analysis, 88–91
portfolio trackers, 143–149
pros and cons of, 223–226
segregated funds, 213
what they invest in, 216–222
where to buy, 214
Mutual Group, The, 64, 70

National Association of Securities Dealers (NASD), 17, 28, 38
Negroponte, Nicholas, 93
Net asset values (NAVs), 139, 217
NetTRADER, 111, 114, 126
New England Funds, 83
News archives, 102–105
on the Internet, 126–129
NewScan, 105, 108
Newsgroups, risks of, *See also* Online fraud, 21
NewsLibrary, 105, 108
No-load mutual funds, *See also* Investment products and Mutual funds, 9, 214–215

Noranda, 122, 158
North American Securities Administrators Association (NASAA), 17, 18, 38, 26, 27
Northern Light Search, 105, 108

Online analysis tools, for mutual funds, *See also* Financial calculators, 47
Online asset mix tools,
for mutual funds, 49–51
general, 51–54
limitations of, 54
Online brokers, 106–107
Online calculators, *See also* Financial calculators, 133
Online company research, 96–107
Online discount brokerages, *See also* Online trading services, 109, 110–111
Online discussion groups, 81
and mutual funds, 91–93
Online education,
about investing, 229–243
cash-based investments, 229–233
Online fraud, 13–21
avoidance of, 26–33
common sources of, 20–21
telltale signs of, 33
types of, 17–21
Online hype, *See also* Online fraud, 28–29
Online information,
about mutual funds, *See also* Mutual funds, 46–48, 82–91
and determining your asset mix, 45–48
and securities regulators, 32–33
company research, 96–107
credibility of, 25
financial search engines, 105–106
government organizations, 106
news archives, 102–105
online trading services, 106–107
validity of, 25, 27–28, 33–38
where to get help, 38
Online information security, 112
Online investing, *See also* Investment planning, Investment products, Online investment planning, 1–6, 109–131
and Canada Savings Bonds, 137–138, 169
and insider information, *See also* Online fraud, 30
and news archives, *See also* Online information, 126–129
and portfolio management, 133–169
and technical problems, 24–25
as a form of gambling, 172
basic concepts of, 197–209
benefits and risks, *See also* Online trading, 7–33, 115–116
cash-based investments, *See also* Investment products, 71–80
commissions and fees, 116–122
discount brokerages, 109, 110–111
in the future, 129–131
integrated software, 161
investment insurance, 113–114
investment product selection, 41–57
monitoring cash-based investments, 134–138
monitoring mutual funds, 138–152
mutual fund commissions, 118–120
mutual funds, 81–93
online trading services, 111–122
security issues, 76–79, 112, 113
services on offer, 114
setting up an account, 114
stocks and bonds, 95–107
what you can buy/sell, 112–113
Online investment planning, 41–57
and asset mix, 56–57
Online investment research, *See also* Online information, 45–48
Online investment tools, 59–69
Online investment tracking, and the future, 162–168
Online news archives, 126–129
Online questionnaires, and asset mix, 49–54
Online research, *See* Online information
Online retirement planning, *See* Retirement planning

INDEX

Online risks, other than fraud, 21–25
Online savings rates, 72–73
Online stock portfolio managers, 158–160
Online stock quotes, 153
Online trading,
  an example of, 122–125
  continuing education, 125
Online trading services, 106–107, 109
  researching, 111–116
Ontario Securities Commission (OSC), 18, 30, 32, 38
Ottawa Citizen, The, 188, 194

PALTrak, 48, 58, 133, 149–152, 169
Pape, Gordon, 143, 191, 194
Pathfinder, 103, 108
Performance measurement, *See* Portfolio management
Phillips, Hager & North, 140, 169, 214, 227
Porta Systems Corp., 100
Portfolio Analytics, 149–152, 169
Portfolio management,
  and Canada Savings Bonds, 137–138
  and mutual funds, 138–152
  and the future, 162–168
  cash-based investments, 134–138
  integrated software programs, 161
  on the Internet, *See also* Online investing, 133–169
  online stock portfolio managers, 158–160
Portfolio management software, 133, 138, 149–152
Portfolio trackers, 133, 138, 143–149
PR Newswire, 104, 108
PricewaterhouseCoopers, 190, 194
Priority Brokerage, 126, 132
Privacy, on the Internet, *See also* Online fraud, 23–24
Pyramid schemes, *See also* Online fraud, 19–20

Quicken, 53, 55, 58, 65, 73, 80, 133, 139, 149, 162–168, 189, 194

Quote.com, 153, 154, 170
QuotesCanada.com, 133, 154, 170

Research, *See* Online investment research
Retirement planning, *See also* Investment planning, Online investment planning
  and financial calculators, 59–69
  and Internet benefits, 9–12
  and Internet risks, 12–33
  five important questions, 60–67
  on the Internet, *See also* Online investing, RRSPs, 175–194
RetireWeb, 66, 70, 178, 194
Reuters MoneyNet, 99, 108
Revenue Canada, 179, 195
Risk scale, 199
Royal Bank Financial Group, 213
Royal Bank of Canada, 36, 38, 74, 76, 80, 86, 113, 125, 132141, 143, 162, 170, 221, 227
RRIFs (Registered Retirement Income Funds), *See also* Investment products, Online investing, Retirement planning, 176, 191–193
RRSPs (Registered Retirement Savings Plans), *See also* Investment products, Online investing, Retirement planning
  and cash-based investments, 71–80
  and income taxes, 65
  and stocks and bonds, 95–107
  calculators, *See* Financial calculators
  on the Internet, 175–194
  self-directed, 96
  what you should know, 186–191

Savings accounts, 205
  and online research, 230–231
Savings rates, and the Internet, 72–73
Saxon Funds, 214, 227
Scam artists, *See also* Online fraud, 13–17

avoidance of, *See also* Online fraud, 31
Scams, exotic, *See also* Online fraud, 19–20
Sceptre Mutual Funds, 214
Schwab, Charles, 172
Scotiabank, 3, 65, 67, 70, 111, 119, 126, 132, 230, 243
Scudder Funds of Canada, 214, 227
Securities and Investments Board, 21
Securities regulators, 32–33
SEDAR (System for Electronic Document Analysis and Retrieval), 46, 106, 108
Segregated funds, 213
Self-directed RRSPs, *See* RRSPs
Selling/buying, on the Internet, *See* Online investing and Online trading services
Seniors Computer Information Project, 179, 195
Shell, Janice, 20
Silicon Investor, 16, 21, 29, 39, 46
Small cap stocks, *See also* Investment products, Stocks, 207–208
SmartMoney, 99, 108, 109, 129, 132
Southam Newspapers, 23, 39, 170
Spam, *See also* Online fraud, 20
Speculative stocks, *See also* Online fraud, 208
Standard and Poor's, 99, 108, 154, 170
Statistics Canada, 3
Steffens, John, 172, 173
Stock portfolio managers, on the Internet, 158–160
Stock quotes,
delayed, 133
on the Internet, 153
real-time, 133
Stock Smart Pro, 99, 108
StockHouse, 95, 99, 102, 108
StockLine, 111
Stockpoint, 154, 159, 170
Stocks, *See also* Investment products, Online investing, 206–208
and online portfolio management, 153–161

and online research, *See also* Online research, 95–107, 238–242
blue chip, 207
emerging growth, 208
large cap, 207
online company research, 96–107
small cap, 207–208
speculative, 208
thinly traded, *See also* Online fraud, 18, 28–29
StockSmart, 160, 170
Strategis, *See also* Industry Canada, 46
Suncor Energy, 102
Sympatico, 66, 236, 243

Talvest Investment Management, 213, 227
Taxes, *See* Income taxes
TDBank Green Line, 113, 117, 126, 132183, 195
Technical problems, on the Internet, 24–25
Telenium, 154, 161, 170
Term deposits, *See also* Investment products, Online investing, 205–206
and online investing, 134
and online research, 232–233
Thinly traded stocks, *See also* Investment products, Online fraud, Stocks, 18, 28–29
Thomson Real Time Quotes, 154, 170
Ticker symbol, 163
Time value of money, 184
Time-Warner, 103
TopFunds, 92, 93
Toronto Stock Exchange (TSE), 29, 39, 91, 148, 239, 243
Trading password, 123
Trailer fee, 118, 120
Trimark, 162, 213, 214, 227

U.K. Financial Services Authority, 39
U.S. Federal Trade Commission, 20
U.S. Securities and Exchange Commission (SEC), 15, 17, 19, 23, 36, 39, 100, 106, 235, 239, 243

INDEX

Validity,
  of online information, 25,
  27–28, 33–38
Vancouver City Savings Credit
  Union, 232, 243
Vancouver Stock Exchange
  (VSE), 29, 39, 46, 239, 243
Vancouver Sun, The, 53, 58, 89,
  93, 149, 170
VERSUS Brokerage, 112, 123

Wall Street Journal, The, 105,
  108, 172
Wall Street Research Net, 95,
  99, 101, 108
Wallman, Steve, 36
Web sites, bogus, *See also*
  Online fraud, 21

Yahoo! Canada, 83, 93, 97, 98,
  108
Young, Duff, 84, 92, 143, 234

ALSO AVAILABLE FROM JIM CARROLL AND RICK BROADHEAD

1999 Canadian Internet Handbook

The 5th anniversary edition of the *Canadian Internet Handbook* focuses on practical information that will help you improve all aspects of your Internet use. Whether you're an experienced Internet user or a novice, you'll find the right tips, tools, and techniques to help you become more efficient online. The *Handbook*'s four themes address the following critical issues:

- Assessing the Effectiveness of Your Web Site — covers everything from online marketing to improving the usability of your site, coupled with valuable design tips from a panel of 17 Canadian "Webmasters"

- Protecting Yourself Online — an in-depth examination of how you can safeguard against viruses, data loss, and hackers

- Improving Your Productivity on the Internet — a review of software that can dramatically improve your productivity; plus numerous techniques that will help you increase the speed of your Internet connection and search the Net faster and more effectively

- Enhancing Your Web Site — shows you how to easily integrate multimedia and e-commerce technologies into your Web site

As a special added bonus, the *1999 Canadian Internet Handbook* includes a free CD-ROM containing trial versions of many of the tools and software programs reviewed in the book. Comprehensive, up-to-date, and designed specifically for Canadians, this high-value resource is truly a "must read" for every Internet user.

$27.95
Available at bookstores across Canada

1999 Canadian Internet Directory and Research Guide

Really two books for the price of one, the *1999 Canadian Internet Directory and Research Guide* gives you the tools you need to maximize your enjoyment and efficiency online.

Written by Canada's bestselling Internet authors, this indispensable guide is essential reading for anyone who's ever tried to find something on the Internet.

You'll learn time-saving techniques and strategies to help you access the information you need in a fraction of the time it currently takes. Of course, part of the challenge in searching the Internet is finding the best places to start. This book highlights and recommends dozens of online search tools that you probably didn't know existed!

The second part of this book contains annotated listings of thousands of Canada's top Internet resources—hand-picked for their content, quality, and usefulness.

$29.95
Available at bookstores across Canada

1999 Canadian Internet New User's Handbook

The *Canadian Internet New User's Handbook* is the bible of Net basics written by Canada's leading Internet experts. It's packed with jargon-free information that demystifies the Net and gets you started—easily and effectively. Completely revised and updated for 1999, the *Canadian Internet New User's Handbook* serves up essential advice that no novice should be without. Key features include:

- a unique cross-country tour of the Internet that demonstrates how Canadians are putting this technology to work
- straightforward instructions on how to plug into the Net, including options for high-speed access
- detailed overviews of the most important Internet tools
- clear, practical explanations of e-mail, the World Wide Web, discussion groups, and interactive services
- valuable tips on how to search for information
- useful insights into how both businesses and individuals can use the Net
- how to set up your own Web site

$16.95

Available at bookstores across Canada

Small Business Online: A Strategic Guide for Canadian Entrepreneurs

If you own or work for a small business, have a home office, or dream of becoming self-employed, this book is for you. *Small Business Online* is the first book of its kind to help Canadian small businesses prosper in this new world of opportunity.

From advice on how to market your Web site to strategies for tackling the Year 2000 problem, *Small Business Online* will show you how to harness the power of the Net to both establish and expand your company. You'll learn how to skillfully use the Internet to:

- assess your entrepreneurial skills
- research a business idea
- formulate a business plan
- obtain financing for your company
- set up your home office
- choose a Web design firm
- gain credibility in the global marketplace
- promote your organization internationally

Loaded with practical, up-to-date advice, this is a book that no small business owner can afford to be without!

$18.95

Available at bookstores across Canada

Good Health Online:
A Wellness Guide for Every Canadian

The amount of health and medical information available on the Internet is nothing less than stunning. But there are many dangers awaiting Canadians seeking health advice on the Net. To help you sort the science from the snake oil, Jim Carroll and Rick Broadhead have prepared this fascinating reference that no Canadian can afford to be without. You will learn how to:

- conduct effective online research into health care matters

- evaluate the credibility of online health information

- avoid the pitfalls of fraudulent, inaccurate or biased information

- deal with Internet-illiterate medical professionals

- assess the dramatic changes that the Internet will bring to the health care industry

Written from a Canadian perspective, *Good Health Online* is ideal for those who want to pursue a healthy lifestyle, research a specific medical topic or use the Internet as a tool for health communication. Whether you're an Internet novice or an expert user, you will find this non-technical book to be a valuable addition to your Internet library. Produced in co-operation with Sympatico.

$16.95

Available at bookstores across Canada

Workshops and Presentations by Rick Broadhead

"Have you ever experienced a presentation that moved so fast and so stretched your picture of how life operates that you knew you'd seen something important, but could barely say what? That happened to me while listening to Internet expert Rick Broadhead.... Rick has co-authored 19 books, including the Canadian Internet Handbook, and he knows his stuff."

Newsletter of the Canadian Association of Professional Speakers, June 1998

Rick Broadhead is acknowledged as one of Canada's leading authorities and public commentators on the Internet. Widely recognized for his extensive industry knowledge and non-technical approach to the Internet, Rick has been retained as a keynote speaker and workshop facilitator by organizations and professional associations across North America.

Rick's expertise has been sought by thousands of professionals in all areas of management, and his consulting services have been used by Fortune 500 companies and other organizations seeking strategic and policy guidance with respect to the Internet and corporate Web site development/management.

His clients include prominent businesses across a wide range of industries, including McDonald's, EMI Music Canada, PolyGram, Manulife Financial, the Royal Bank of Canada, Imperial Oil, Sprint Canada, Mackenzie Financial Services, BC TEL, CTV Television, Microsoft, and VISA International, where he was commissioned to prepare an overview of the strategic implications of the Internet for VISA's member financial institutions worldwide. In addition, his services have been used by a wide variety of associations and membership organizations, including the Canadian Real Estate Association, the Canadian Paint and Coatings Association, the National Utility Contractors Association, the Canadian Wood Council, the Canadian Association of Insurance and Financial Advisors, the Canadian Meat Council, Credit Union Central of Canada, and the Municipal Electric Association.

Rick is also an instructor at York University's Division of Executive Development in Toronto, where he has advised executives and senior managers from hundreds of leading North American firms and helped them to integrate the Internet into all facets of their businesses.

For further information about Rick Broadhead's consulting and speaking services, you may contact him directly by telephone at 416-487-5220 or by e-mail at **rickb@sympatico.ca**. Alternatively, for speaking engagements, you may contact his representatives at CanSpeak Presentations using the numbers listed below. They will be pleased to assist you!

1-800-561-3591 (Central and Eastern Canada)
1-800-665-7376 (Western Canada)

For more detailed information about Rick Broadhead, please visit his Web site:
www.rickbroadhead.com

Need to Prepare Your Organization for the New Millennium?

Jim Carroll — Canada's Leading Futurist

"You are a masterful presenter….. you certainly opened a lot of eyes very wide in the audience. You did it in a charming and engaging way, and you greatly increased the knowledge of everyone in attendance."

David Peterson, former Premier of Ontario

Let's face it — something big is happening. The so-called "information age" is causing dramatic and substantial change in our personal and working lives. Yet making sense of the implications of a society and economy that are increasingly wired together has been a challenge — until now.

Jim Carroll, C.A., has dazzled tens of thousands of North Americans with a keynote speech, seminar or workshop that focuses on the change being wrought on our social, economic and business systems as a result of the emergence of what he calls "the wired world."

No less an authority than *The Financial Post* commented that he is *"one of the most in-demand speakers"* in the country, leaving no doubt that he can help your organization prepare for the dramatic change that will occur with the new millennium . . . in a presentation that will enthrall you.

That's why organizations large and small, such as the World Congress of Association Executives, the Conference Board of Canada, the Royal Bank, the Canadian Construction Association, the Governments of Canada and Ontario, Stentor, Scotia MacLeod, Ontario Hospital Association, Nortel, CIBC, Montreal Trust, IBM, Remax, the Canadian Home Builders Association, the Canadian Community Newspaper Association and others have sought the views of Mr. Carroll in order to prepare for the future.

For an extensive list of clients and other background information on Mr. Carroll, visit his Web site at **www.jimcarroll.com**. Contact him by phone at 905-855-2950 or by e-mail at **jcarroll@jimcarroll.com**. A video of his speeches is available online and on CD-ROM.

For more information on booking Jim Carroll, call:
THE NATIONAL SPEAKERS BUREAU
IN CANADA 1-800-661-4110
INTERNATIONAL AND USA 1-604-734-3663
FAX 1-604-734-8906
INTERNET speakers@nsb.com/www.nsb.com